A Longer Life

H. Beric Wright, MB, FRCS
and Alan Bailey, MB, MRCP
BUPA MEDICAL CENTRE

Blackie: Glasgow and London

Published by Blackie and Son Limited
Bishopbriggs, Glasgow G64 2NZ
450/452 Edgware Road, London W2 IEG

©BUPA Medical Research and Development Limited 1976
First published 1976

(ISBN 0 216 90142 1)

Filmset in Ireland by Doyle Photosetting Ltd., Tullamore
Printed in Great Britain by Robert MacLehose & Co. Ltd.,
15 Foulis Street, Anniesland, Glasgow

Contents

Preface to the series

The medical profession has long been brought up to genuflect at the altar of preventive medicine, but if an average patient were to go to an equally average—and possibly non-existent—GP to ask either for a health check, or the more simple question 'How am I, doctor?', he would, more likely than not, get a dusty answer. Equally, if the same patient (i.e. the consumer of health care), having got this dusty answer, then took himself off for a health check, had the results sent to his doctor and then went back for interpretation and advice, the chances still are that he would not be received with much enthusiasm. Knowing the likelihood of this reception, had the health check centre said, 'Look, Mr. Robinson, your blood pressure is a bit high at X, your cholesterol raised at Y, etc.—do go and see your doctor about it', the doctor might still be resentful: neither patient nor health check can win.

Although traditionally doctors are taught the merits of prevention and the virtues of health education, their basic conversion is only just beginning. Of course, public health measures have improved, mother and baby clinics flourish, mass radiography has been accepted and so on, but the concept of trying to persuade patients to avoid disease and the attempt to pick up early signs of disease before the changes have caused symptoms—called presymptomatic diagnosis—is relatively new. And, to be fair, it is only recently that preventive medicine has had anything much to offer in the way of effective treatment.

When I started in this work in 1958, some regarded me as a dangerous heretic for advocating the treatment of raised blood pressure (hypertension) in the middle-aged. Now, although there is legitimate disagreement about precisely when, or at what levels in relation to age, treatment should be instigated, there is agreement that some raised blood pressures should be treated in order to reduce the chances of long-term harm or to postpone death.

Similarly, the treatment of raised blood fats (lipids, cholesterol) is in the same phase as blood pressure was a decade or so ago. In another five years, I believe that its treatment will be as commonplace as the treatment of hypertension is now.

Unfortunately, the statistics of justifying such treatment are very

i

complex and expensive. Comparable groups of several hundred treated and untreated people need to be studied and followed-up over five or ten years, or even longer. Additionally, patients' attitudes and behaviour alter by their mere involvement in an experiment. Nevertheless, at this time, there is an epidemic of coronary heart disease (CHD) attacking and killing thousands of middle-aged men each year and there are good theoretical grounds for believing that the identification and treatment of vulnerable people is the only way of reducing this death toll.

As with blood pressure, there is a growing body of evidence that treating some of the coronary risk factors, like reducing weight, stopping smoking and bringing down cholesterol, does in practice reduce coronary risk. That prevention is worthwhile for CHD is still an act of faith we freely admit—but it does seem sensible, it is feasible and it apparently does no harm. For these and other reasons we at the British United Provident Association Medical Centre are strongly in favour of it.

Again, going back to our early experience of 'health checks', it used to be said, particularly by doctors, 'Why go to that place? They will only tell you, you are too fat and smoke too much, and you know that.' In addition, the doctors would further complain that there was a great undesirable danger that people would be encouraged to worry about their health and have their hypochondria pandered to. Some of this may be true, but hypochondria never killed anybody and coronary thrombosis and breast cancer do.

This series of booklets is based on the following beliefs:
1. That common and killing conditions like CHD and breast cancer can only be begun to be dealt with by presymptomatic diagnosis.

2. That regular health screening, which is to be regarded as preventive maintenance on people, will help this. You do not wait until your teeth ache to have them looked at and, if necessary, filled. In addition, you do not know what your blood pressure is, how your liver is standing up to the strain of what you eat and drink, unless the indices are measured. Further, it is much easier to assess the significance of a change found today, if one knows

what the measurement was a year or two back. There is over-whelming support for everyone having a medical log book or 'vital profile'.

3. That people are more likely to react sensibly if they know what their indices are and ought to be and the reasons for bringing them back to normal.

CHD is, to a degree, a disease of over-indulgence and indiscipline. Anything that we or anyone else can do to make overweight people eat less, sedentary people take exercise, cigarette smokers give up, stressed people sort themselves out, and so on, is, in our view, well worthwhile. Preventive medicine hinges largely round health education—altering attitudes and behaviour. Health education may be less exciting than running an intensive care unit and bathroom scales may be unglamorous compared with a scalpel, but the unexciting will keep more people alive.

Our fourth belief then, is that people can be persuaded to mend their ways and live more sensibly. Hopefully, if they do this, they will be both happier and live longer. We cannot prove it, but it does seem sensible.

These then are a series of health education booklets, written by the staff of a medical unit dedicated to preventive medicine. They are aimed at the two commonest killing diseases of men and women: coronary heart disease and breast cancer. But they also discuss other things, cover other ground and raise wider issues, we hope in an interesting and helpful way. Some of the views expressed are controversial and are included to promote discussion and provoke interest. Because of this, it must be said that they represent the views of the writers and not necessarily the official policy of BUPA.

BUPA is a sickness insurance company which believes that prevention can be better than cure, which is why it set up the Medical Centre in 1970. Its faith has been justified at least by the support of the public. In 1974, over 20,000 people paid to come to the centre, because they thought that some form of health check was worthwhile. We hope for the day when health maintenance will be an accepted part of the health service: when this happens it will be a 'health' and not a 'sickness' service.

The booklets are designed as a family, but each one covers a separate topic and to that extent at least, should be able to stand on its own.

Basic Health Maintenance

Booklet 1 gives an introduction to the philosophy and technology of health screening and outlines some of the benefits likely to accrue from regular maintenance. (ISBN 0 216 90138 3)

Heart Disease

Booklet 2 is concerned with the main coronary risk factors and how to deal with some of them. (ISBN 0 216 90139 1)

Fitness Without Fantasies

Booklet 3 is about living sensibly in terms of diet, weight control, exercise and smoking. (ISBN 0 216 90140 5)

A Woman's Life

Booklet 4 is for and about women. But it covers more than minor gynaecology and breast cancer. It tries—admittedly through the eyes of a male—to look at some of the social and psychological problems that women face in today's world. (ISBN 0 216 90141 3)

My colleagues and I hope that you will find the series both interesting and helpful. We would welcome your views and comments and we thank the publishers for bullying us into doing the writing and then producing the booklets.

London 1975

H. B. Wright

1
Basic Health Maintenance

Alan Bailey, MB, MRCP

Introduction

As medicine advances the pattern of disease changes. Medicine has to continue to advance to keep up with it. Medical manpower is expensive to train and costly to maintain. Its knowledge is enormous. In order for people to benefit from modern medicine they have to be put in contact with the right man. Until recently patients only contacted the doctor when they felt ill—often too late for a cure to be effective. But we need to strive towards the World Health Organisation's definition of health—that is, a complete feeling of mental and physical well-being. Doctors may never achieve this, but it must be their aim. At present, little more than lip service is paid towards preventive medicine in Britain. British management is aware of the problems of health and disease in industry and has made possible the establishment of the first computerised Medical Centre in Europe, under the auspices of the Institute of Directors and the British United Provident Association. With more than ten years of experience of screening and counselling more than 70,000 men and women from industry, in an increasingly efficient and sophisticated way, the Medical Centre has been asked to 'write up' its philosophy and findings in a comprehensible form for the people who use it.

This first booklet traces the changes in medicine over the years that have produced a new approach to medical care. It examines briefly the statistics by which much medicine is judged today. Finally, it describes the present state of the art of comprehensive health maintenance through screening, illustrating the text with figures and case histories—anonymous medical stories to illustrate the facts.

Historical Aspects

Our starting point in this study is a case history, that of Thomas Parr, now long since dead so he need not remain anonymous. Thomas Parr was a farmworker on the agricultural estate of the Earl of Arundel and came to his landlord's attention in 1635, when he was reputed to have achieved the great age of 152, this being quite a remarkable age for that time when life expectancy was probably only thirty years. The Earl had him removed to London and exhibited him for all to see in a pub in the Strand called The Queen's Tavern. The poor man only lasted six weeks, during which time he was presented to the King, Charles I. Because of this, the post mortem was carried out by the King's physician, the father of modern medicine, William Harvey, who reports first on the cause of death:

> The cause of death seemed fairly referrible to a sudden change in the non-naturals, the chief mischief being connected with the change of air, which through the whole course of life had been inhaled of perfect purity,—light, cool, and mobile, whereby the praecordia and lungs were more freely ventilated and cooled; but in this great advantage, in this grand cherisher of life this city (London) is especially destitute; a city whose grand characteristic is an immense concourse of men and animals, and where ditches abound, and filth and offal lie scattered about, to say nothing of the smoke engendered by the general use of sulphureous coal as fuel, whereby the air is at all times rendered heavy, but much more so in the autumn than at any other season. Such an atmosphere could not have been found otherwise than insalubrious to one coming from the open, sunny and healthy region of Salop; it must have been especially so to one already aged and infirm.

and then, on the evidence of the post mortem examination, that he had indeed achieved a great age:

> The organs of generation were healthy, the penis neither retracted nor extenuated, nor the scrotum filled with any serious infiltration, as happens so commonly among the decrepit; the

1.4

testes, too, were sound and large; so that it seemed not improbable that the common report was true, viz. that he did public penance under a conviction for incontinence, after he had passed his hundredth year; and his wife, whom he had married as a widow in his hundred-and-twentieth year, did not deny that he had intercourse with her after the manner of other husbands with their wives, nor until about twelve years back had he ceased to embrace her frequently.

Alas, undoubtedly a victim of the environment. An environment which everyone agrees man has improved but in doing so has brought upon himself different kinds of problems. To illustrate this it is necessary to study the pattern of disease from Thomas Parr's time up until the present.

For the next two hundred years the documentation of medical events was not good. It was the era of quacks, sham medicine, bleeding, purges, amputations and extreme poverty. An attempt at some order was made by the establishment of such institutions as the Royal College of Physicians in 1518 and the Society of Apothecaries in 1617, who would issue licences to doctors who practiced reasonably straight medicine, but it was not until the beginning of the nineteenth century, when man started to observe the interreaction between himself and the environment, that the great discoveries which began to alter the pattern of disease were made. Epidemiology, which is the science of looking at people, rather than individuals, in relationship to their environment and their disease, was probably born with the work of John Snow.

John Snow was one of the first students to qualify from the new school of medicine in Newcastle in the 1820s and eventually became an anaesthetist at the Westminster Hospital in London. He is probably best remembered for having successfully given chloroform to Queen Victoria during the birth of one of her children in 1853. At that time London was in the clutches of one of the most severe cholera epidemics ever recorded. During an epidemic in Soho in 1854 there were over 500 deaths in a week. No-one knew the cause, there was no cure for it and it was rapidly fatal. John Snow believed, and it was a belief, that the germ that was causing the disease was carried in the drinking water and during the evenings he would mark on a map of central

London the houses where cholera deaths had occurred. He eventually came to the conclusion that the common factor between all the cholera deaths in Soho was a water pump in Broad Street. John Snow wrote to the Westminster Council, who were responsible for the water supply, and asked that it be discontinued and gave his theories as to why. Westminster Council pointed out that if the water supply was stopped everybody would die of dehydration. The story goes that John Snow had to go out and dismantle the pump himself in order to prove his theory, with the result that cholera was more or less eradicated from that part of London. Later it was discovered that a large sewer was draining into the well that supplied the Broad Street pump. In 1883 the cholera germ was seen for the first time under the microscope and the missing link, the connection between John Snow's theories and the result of his preventive practice, was demonstrated. Around this time, the middle of the nineteenth century, a government department in England started to collect statistics on how many people died, how old they were, what they died of, when they died etc. and Figure 1a shows how the pattern of death since this time has dramatically altered.

During the Victorian era the great killers were tuberculosis, smallpox, diphtheria, cholera, typhoid; in fact all infectious diseases. Diseases due to germs (bacteria), too small for the naked eye to see, gained access to the human body through the mouth or nose, or in the food or water that was consumed. Gradually, these micro-organisms were detected and systematically eradicated. Firstly by prevention; that is either by making the human being resistant to the effects of the germ, such as smallpox vaccination, or by cleanliness (in other words, when a germ cannot be eradicated you avoid eating the food contaminated by it or breathing the air that harbours it). Secondly by drugs; medicine designed specifically to kill the germs. Tuberculosis provides a good example of this sort of disease which streptomycin, invented in 1944, has almost eradicated. (Interestingly tuberculosis itself was already on the wane as Figure 1b demonstrates. The early reduction in the number of cases of tuberculosis reported before antibiotic therapy was available is almost certainly due to improved sanitation and public health measures, examined in more detail later.)

During the first half of this century man's life expectancy gradually increased and specific cures were discovered for some diseases.

1.6

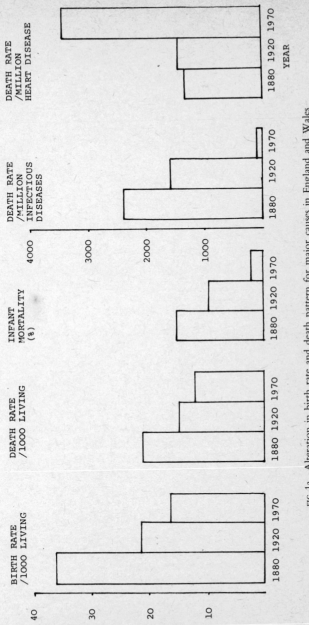

FIG 1a Alteration in birth rate and death pattern for major causes in England and Wales 1880–1970 (Registrar General)

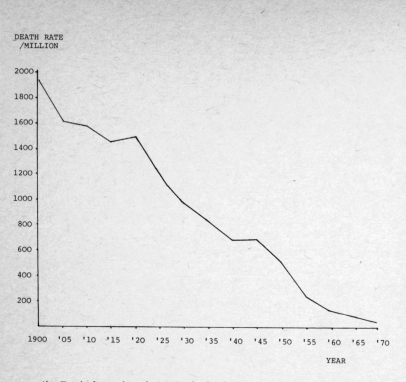

DEATH RATE
/MILLION

FIG 1b   Deaths from tuberculosis in England and Wales 1900–70 (Registrar General)

Pernicious anaemia—nearly always fatal—turned out to be due to a simple vitamin deficiency. Diabetes, on the other hand, was discovered to be the complex manifestation of a deficiency in an important hormone called insulin, discovered in 1922 and first extracted shortly afterwards. In 1927 a question appeared in the Specialist examination of the Royal College of Physicians, probably the most difficult medical exam in the country, on a disease called ischaemic heart disease. Few candidates then had heard of it; now almost fifty years later, it is the scourge of the civilised world. Also at that time the motor car was the fashionable thing to have, a few rich people owned one. Now it causes 4000 deaths a week world-wide. Lung cancer was practically unknown in women and it was very rare to see a woman smoke; now we are predominantly a smoking nation, lung cancer a

1.8

cruel and speedy death for which, once established, only palliative remedies are available. It kills one man in Britain every twenty minutes and is rapidly becoming one of the major causes of death in women. Life expectancy in the last twenty-five years of 'affluent' nationalised medicine and the welfare state has increased by little more than a year, and twenty-eight million prescriptions for tranquillisers and anti-depressants were prescribed in 1972; so much for the quality of life.

Comprehensive Health Screening

The pattern of death in the 1970s is given in Figure 1c. By far the commonest cause is disease of the heart and blood vessels (and the figures given apply to the 35–64 age-group). Unfortunately, the commonest single presentation of a heart attack is sudden death, and this occurs before any medical help has arrived. Much the same applies to strokes, due to hardening of the arteries to the brain: even if not immediately fatal there is little that medical treatment can offer.

The pattern of disease (as distinct from death) is shown in Figure 1d from a recent survey carried out by the Royal College of General Practitioners. This shows that attendance in general practice, apart from minor coughs and colds, centres around 'stress'-induced disease. Stress is an expression that has its origins in physics and until recently it was more of a technical than a medical term. Now we use it as a measure of man's interaction with his environment. Everyone experiences stress from day to day, and mostly this is normal. At times the stress factor becomes too great, leading to physical and psychological manifestations. Increased stress may contribute to depression, heart disease, ulcers and a host of other symptoms and diseases for which no simple physical cause can be found. Symptoms of early stress may be headaches, pains in the chest, indigestion, palpitations, muscle and joint pains, looseness of the bowels and so on. The presence of these symptoms in turn leads to worry and introspection

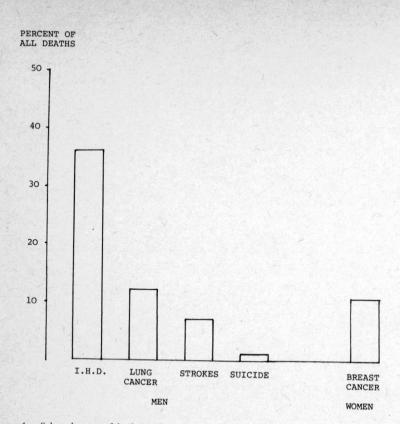

PERCENT OF
ALL DEATHS

FIG 1c   Selected causes of death (aged 35–64) in England and Wales 1972 (Registrar General)
(I.H.D. = Ischaemic Heart Disease)

about one's health, an increase in smoking habit, alcohol consumption, irritability and shortness of temper with colleagues at work, rows at home, setting up a vicious circle which will lead, if not interrupted, to one of the serious manifestations mentioned above.

To combat the causes of death and disease in the middle-aged population it is necessary through a comprehensive medical system to detect disease at the earliest point in time. This process is called screening. It has been used successfully for most of this century to combat disease. Mass X-rays, a public health measure introduced in the 1930s, were designed to detect lung conditions, particularly tuber-

1.10

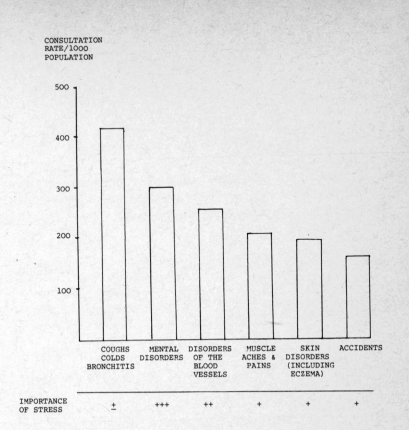

FIG 1d   Consultation rates in general practice for selected disorders and stress rating (RCGP 1974)

culosis and pneumoconiosis in miners, before the patient was aware that he had the disease, so that treatment was instituted early and, therefore more effectively. In the case of tuberculosis, the patient was isolated during the infectious phase so he did not pass the disease on. As has been shown already, these measures and a general increase in the standard of living produced a fall in the incidence of tuberculosis long before anti-tuberculous drugs were introduced.

In industry much simple screening is carried out. Sight tests are performed on drivers of public service vehicles; heart tests for airline pilots; bacterial examinations for food handlers to check that they do not harbour any dangerous germs that might be transmitted. For the general public, since the 1950s, cervical smear tests have.been available to detect early cancer of the womb, and all new-born children are screened for a rare and correctible genetic deficiency called phenyl-ketonuria which, untreated, produces severe mental and physical retardation.

These rather specialised examples of individual screening procedures can all be combined and expanded to produce a comprehensive screening system (the Americans call it multiphasic screening) which is designed to look at all the body systems, regardless of whether the patient is aware of anything wrong or not. It is similar to having the car regularly serviced and it allows the best possible chance of treatment being successful. Moreover, it is possible through such a system to identify areas of stress or 'stress vulnerability'. Analysis of the results is used to improve the system's efficiency at detection and increase our knowledge of the natural history of disease. Because so much of the screening procedure is based on statistical analysis—a word about statistics, before examining the results.

Statistics

Statistics are usually based on a sample of people and before conclusions can be interpreted in general one must be sure that the sample is not biased. For example, if you want to study blood pressure in people with heart disease, an obvious place to go is into a ward of a big hospital, where on every medical ward you will find patients suffering from heart disease. Moreover, you would find several patients suffering from disease other than of the heart and it would be quite simple to compare statistically measurements in one group with the same measurements in the other group. The results, however, would not be representative of people in general who have heart disease, for the people who are sitting in a hospital bed do not represent the full spectrum of heart disease. They do not, for instance, represent the people who have died of heart disease nor do they represent the people who have yet to have their heart disease diagnosed. Some modern medical treatment is based on statistical studies of samples which are not representative of the disease in general.

The next trap for the unwary in interpreting statistics is the assumption that the relationship between two statistics represents anything more than chance. Too often one measurement is assumed to cause the change in another, and statistics are sometimes misinterpreted because causality is assumed. Recently a psychiatrist demonstrated a statistical relationship between certain types of fingerprints and neuroticism. There is, however, no suggestion that the fingerprint is the cause of the neuroticism, nor indeed that to remove the fingertips would be effective treatment for neuroticism. However, in every walk of life today one can hear and read advice from 'experts' based on misinterpretations of statistical relationships.

Finally, when examining the changes in pattern of disease, an increase in the incidence will often have three components. Firstly, there is a true increase due to the disease becoming commoner. Secondly, methods of diagnosing may be improving, and the apparent increase in the incidence only represents an increased efficiency in detection (greater sensitivity). Thirdly, the increase may be due to the fact that people are living longer and the disease has a preference for higher age-groups. As we will see later, the increase in incidence of heart disease consists of all three components.

1.13

The Screening Process

In order for the Medical Centre to be able to screen as many people as possible a small computer co-ordinates its activities. The purpose of the computer is to collect together as many facts about the patient as possible and present them to the doctor in a rapid and understandable way. Non-medical but specially trained people, usually nurses, apply a test to a subject, press a button, and the computer reads and stores the results. Later specialists examine and interpret X-rays and cardiographs and report to the computer; and blood is drawn and analysed. During his visit the patient is questioned, by a system of slides run by the computer, about his working life, social and physical habits, past and present medical history and all the facts are collected and printed out on a report for the doctor who sees and examines the patient. He checks the results and takes any necessary steps to correct abnormalities, where possible. It has long been appreciated that the conventional medical technique of waiting for the patient to come to the doctor is only scratching the iceberg of physical disease present in the community.

The results of the Medical Centre's examinations may be divided into three groups. First there is the clear-cut presymptomatic diagnosis. Here the patient is either unaware that disease is present or it has not been detected by the medical system previously. They include heart disease (7·4%), digestive disorders (2·4%), prostate and urine troubles (1·1%), lung disease (1%), skin and bone problems (2·1%), cancer (0·2%), piles, varicose veins, and other miscellaneous problems (7%). In fact, nearly a fifth of the patients fall into this category—some may have more than one diagnosis made. This is straightforward clinical medicine at the detection stage and arrangements are made, through the patient's doctor, for the condition to be treated.

The next group contains those people who are not actually diseased but medical experience tells us that the probability of developing a particular disease is high. The prediction is made for a group rather than an individual and the individual is allocated to the group. The statistical experience is that of the group, and the preventitive aspect of the exercise comes in attempting to move the high-risk group individual into a lower-risk group—on the same basis that it is safer to walk on the pavement than in the middle of the road, and we should try to prevent people doing the latter. (However, occasionally a pavement-walker will be killed and some of the middle-of-the-road-walkers will survive.) The measurements that predict rather than diagnose are weight, blood pressure, blood fat (cholesterol) levels, lung function tests and so on. From the personal profile come habits such as smoking and drinking, early symptoms such as pain or sputum production, and an account of past and familial illnesses. All these factors combine together to predict the possible development of disease (dealt with more fully in the next booklet with regard to coronary risk factors). If one examines just three of these factors—the blood pressure, cholesterol level, and the smoking habit—and groups individuals into six groups according to their coronary risk, it is found that only a small proportion of our 'healthy' population fall into the top group (about eight per 1000) but of these, half are found to have an abnormal cardiograph indicating that heart disease is already present. The number of individuals falling into the next two categories is about thirteen per cent, and although established heart disease is unusual, their risk of developing it may be ten times greater than individuals at the other end of the scale. Here is an exciting development in medical practice, which, as it becomes more accurate, will allow us to identify the individuals for preventative advice.

The final section of identifiable individuals are those whose personality and personal habits identify them as stress-vulnerable. Here the computer interview covers areas of home, work and personal habits in a private and objective manner. On the subject of work, the stress areas covered are holidays, travelling and driving habits, job description, responsibility and security. Areas of home life covered include family rows and worries, sexual activity and happiness of marriage. General questions about satisfaction with life, lack of confidence, ability to make decisions, sleep habits and a variety of psychosomatic symptoms complete an overall picture of the individual ready for a doctor's interpretation and advice.

Examples of the general stress questions are as follows with the percentage responding positively indicated:

1. Are you unusually worried, tense or anxious?
                                        —Yes response 25%

2. Do you get irritable or bad tempered?

—Yes response 34%

3. Do you feel run down or lacking in energy or have unusual tiredness or fatigue?

—Yes response 30%

4. Do you feel unusually 'fed up' or depressed?

—Yes response 22%

More significant than the number of positive responders to the individual questions are the number who answer positively more than one (34%) and more than two (14%).

Here in the last group one is beginning to identify the patient at risk. With these and other questions, and by continual feed-back of the results and doctors' opinions of the findings, the detection system is monitored and improved.

Case Histories

To clarify in an individual way the three categories of patients benefiting from the comprehensive screening system, six case histories will assist.

Case 1

A bright young man in his late thirties, working for large public corporation, is nearing the top of the ladder. At routine screening he complained of piles for many years, 'not serious enough to bother the doctor about'. However, the examination revealed that a small but chronic blood loss from these piles had thinned his blood to 50%. Three weeks away from work and a simple operation restored it to 100%. Afterwards, the patient realised that for a year or two he had been slowing down, so imperceptibly that he had not noticed, although his employers had and were worried that he would not make the top after a promising start. This case demonstrates the simplicity of the art. Piles are extremely common and painful, yet only a small proportion of patients seek advice. Unless asked and encouraged they spend years of misery, being reminded of their condition every time they sit down.

Case 2

This illustrates the more complex patient: a forty-year-old man, the pilot of an executive jet of a large multi-national corporation. He was found to have raised blood pressure, raised blood fat level and minor abnormalities on his cardiograph. He had an aggressive personality, smoked heavily and was overweight. He was, undoubtedly, most unsuited for his occupation and he and his company were advised (with his permission) that he should not be piloting a plane. Unfortunately, this patient died suddenly while on holiday two months after the examination and initiation of treatment. If his first screening had been sooner he might be alive today.

Case 3

Figure 1e tells the story of a regularly screened businessman. Examinations on him were carried out aged 45, 47, 51 and 53 years and the upper line shows the cholesterol level on each occasion. The lower line is the mean (average) for each year. The cholesterol level is the most precise of many factors for predicting heart disease. This patient began above par and the divergent pattern is alarming and has now been corrected by diet alone (although he may need tablets in the future). The patient has no physical symptoms, but his father died suddenly in his fifties of heart disease. Although a 'one-off' screening examination is useful, the 'three-dimensional' picture illustrated here is of even greater value.

Case 4

A fifty-five-year-old man, in a highly technical, over-stressed and

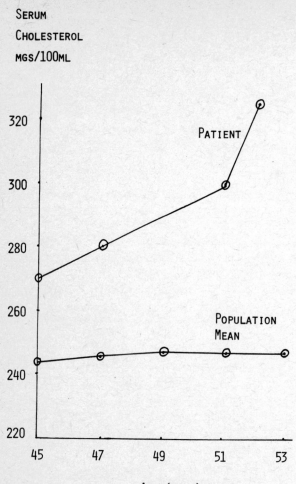

SERUM
CHOLESTEROL
MGS/100ML

PATIENT

POPULATION
MEAN

AGE (YRS.)

FIG 1e   Serum cholesterol measurement over an eight-year period in one patient compared with the mean (BUPA Medical Centre)

1.18

responsible job which he had managed well for fifteen years. At routine screening he scored highly on the stress scores and complained of an increase in smoking and, particularly, drinking habit. Blood tests confirmed that he was drinking too much, but follow-up of the stress lead showed him to be on the verge of a nervous breakdown. He was admitted to hospital the day after screening, before the crisis, and made a full and uneventful recovery. Had his nervous collapse occurred at work, lives would almost certainly have been lost.

Four cases demonstrating the different types of problem occurring in around one third of those attending the Medical Centre.

In addition to the problems that the system is designed to detect it also makes discoveries that have slipped through the net elsewhere. Any diagnostic unit will be able to produce such case histories—and the next two are not meant to imply criticism of the existing health services.

Case 5

A fifty-year-old lorry driver who had been under treatment from his family doctor for depression for six months decided, on reading about the Medical Centre, to spend money on a second opinion. Part of the examination, an X-ray, showed that he had a rare disease of the bones and the reason for his depression was that too much calcium (detected on the blood test) was being released by the diseased bones and circulating in the blood. Treatment of the underlying bone disease and the high blood calcium quickly restored the patient's mental state to normal. It is not often realised by the public that abnormal psychological behaviour may be related to a correctible physical disorder, and it is important—and indeed standard psychiatric practice—to ensure that no such disease exists before treating depression and other forms of mental illness.

Case 6

A fifty-four-year-old managing director had complained of palpitations for many years. As a young man he used to wake in the night to find his heart beating rapidly. At that time he was fully investigated

(1950s) and treated with a mild sedative (a barbiturate). After some years he ceased to be followed-up by the hospital and obtained a supply of tablets regularly from his local doctor. For some months prior to his first routine visit to the Medical Centre he thought the palpitations had become a little worse and had increased his dose of barbiturate, which he had been on for nearly twenty years—and which are habit forming and sometimes addictive. At his examination an abnormal heart rhythm was detected for which more modern treatment was now available and in fact had been for several years. The patient has now been weaned off barbiturates and is palpitation-free. This case history stresses the importance of regular check-ups in patients who are on long-term treatment, to monitor its effect and to alter it in the light of new discoveries and additional disease.

The Research Angle

Modern medicine would be more powerful if more was known about the natural history of disease. Some diseases have a short life such as measles or pneumonia. Measles has a natural history thus: the measles virus enters the body in a breath of air that has been contaminated by a measles sufferer. Once absorbed it spends a week or more setting up a reaction inside the body and after about two weeks a massive fight takes place between the poison of the virus and the body's defence mechanism, which results in the typical features of measles. The body defences nearly always win—the skin and other areas heal up (occasionally leaving the scars of the battle)—and the patient, because he has built up his defences during this attack, is protected for life from further attacks. The illness probably only lasts three or four weeks and is rarely life-threatening (although complications like deafness, as a result of part of the battle taking place in the delicate part of the ear, do occur).

An entirely different problem exists in the study of the natural history of heart disease or some other illness which is not caused by a single factor—such as the measles virus—but seems to be the result of a combination of factors (the epidemiologist calls this multifactorial). For fighting and preventing such a disease, more knowledge is necessary, and there is no doubt that considerable pathology takes place before the patient is aware of the sickness. Figure 1f is a hypothetical representation of the natural history of a multifactorial disease and the levels in which study and intervention (treatment or prevention) may be made. Note that the clinical phase of the disease—i.e. when it is

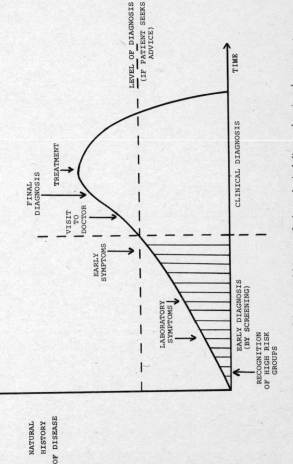

FIG 1f Representation of the natural history of a hypothetical disease showing the stages at which diagnosis may be made

likely that it will present itself to the patient and/or doctor—is late on in its natural history. Before that phase there are various methods of detecting it, but the patient will not regard himself as ill. Only by encouraging the patient to submit to regular examinations will the precursors of the disease be detected—and the course of the disease plotted. This is illustrated in a real disease like coronary artery disease. We know little at present of the natural history of the disease. Pathologists have noticed 'fatty streaks' being deposited on the inside of young people's blood vessels at an early age. This might be the start of atheroma, yet through puberty they seem to disappear. Severe atheroma, however, was seen in the arteries of pilots—all young men—killed in the Vietnam war, compared with civilians of the same age dying from other causes. This raises the question—Is this the start of a generalised process or was its deposition related to the stress of war? The physiologist has studied the circulation that keeps the heart fuelled and has found it to be different from all other circulations in that it fills when the heart is relaxed, whereas other arteries fill when the heart is contracted. All these facts and many others (referred to here and in a later booklet) have helped to piece together the natural history of coronary artery disease, but it is similar to trying to piece together a jig-saw with pieces from many different puzzles—and still the majority of pieces are missing. In other words we are nowhere near being able to describe the life history of coronary artery disease in the same terms as measles.

Research at the Medical Centre will assist in defining the natural history of various multifactorial diseases. To do this we borrow a concept from the ancient Roman Army—the cohort. A cohort is a group of soldiers who are sent out to fight and go on fighting until they are all dead or defeated—they are not replaced by reinforcements—although another cohort may be sent to assist. In the medical sense the use of the word is similar—a cohort of people attending the Medical Centre is selected and they go about their daily work fighting disease and environment just like anyone else. Some will die over the years, the others will be regularly screened for signs of disease or its precursors. The dead people are not replaced in the study group but after some years a comparison is made between the survivors and those who have died, and the results of the regular examinations are analysed in an attempt to map out parts of the life

1.22

story of the disease. It is only by being able to make up a cohort of healthy people and examining them regularly, that such an exercise is possible. But the results will take time—maybe as long as the disease takes to manifest itself—and the work is complex and fastidious. Luckily with a sophisticated computer system at present being developed, much of the work is simplified.

The Middle-Aged Woman

So unhealthy are middle-aged men that, by the time both sexes have reached fifty, there are four times as many widows as widowers. This difference is largely due to the men's excessive death rate from heart disease. But for the women this is also a dangerous age. Firstly, the mortality experience of woman is approaching that of man, the death rate from lung cancer, and heart disease is rising rapidly (Figure 1g). This is to some extent due to the women adopting the men's bad habits of smoking, working in unhealthy environments and thus taking less exercise and experiencing more stress. Although their hormonal constitution will probably continue to protect them from hardening of the arteries and heart disease, women would be wise to look now at the philosophy described for men.

Secondly, there is the problem of breast cancer. In the 35–64 age-group breast cancer is responsible for more than a tenth of the deaths, and the incidence is rising. Treatment has altered little in sixty years and the results of treatment are related to the stage of the disease rather than the nature of the treatment—the earlier the disease is detected and treated, the better the outcome. Moreover, if the cancer is small enough, a simple, non-mutilating operation may be possible, rather than mastectomy (removal of the whole breast). Using modern techniques, including on occasions a special type of breast X-ray, cancerous growths the size of a small pea can be detected, but only if the breasts are regularly checked. The Medical Centre has screened over 12,000 women, many of whom return annually, and has detected some ninety early cancers a rate of just over seven per 1000 patients

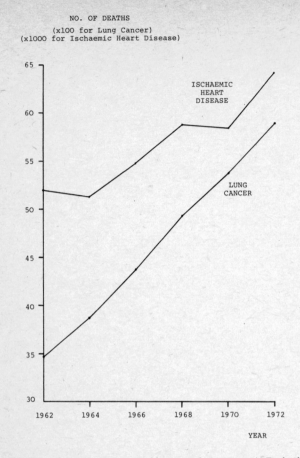

NO. OF DEATHS

(x100 for Lung Cancer)
(x1000 for Ischaemic Heart Disease)

ISCHAEMIC
HEART
DISEASE

LUNG
CANCER

YEAR

FIG 1g   Death (all ages) from lung cancer and heart attacks in women in England and Wales 1962–72 (Registrar General)

examined. Luckily, nine out of ten lumps or abnormalities in the breast turn out not to be cancerous, but they have to be checked carefully just the same, and the patient reassured. It is ironic that in Britain so much emphasis is placed on screening for cancer of the cervix, when breast cancer is more than four times commoner and on the increase.

Finally, the late forties and fifties are the menopausal years, and

1.24

many women need particular understanding at this time as a marked psychological and physiological change of life overtakes them. There is a dearth of good advice about what to expect, what is normal and what mental and physical adjustments may be necessary. During these years and onwards the incidence of depression rises, often this presents insidiously and goes undetected. These women are not 'ill', but they need help and understanding, or put another way, preventive maintenance. This is even more important when women, in this fiercly competitive world, are holding down responsible senior jobs.

Conclusion

This introductory booklet has attempted to explain the philosophy and scientific thinking behind a new form of medicine: the practice of looking ahead, anticipating illness and rooting it out before it becomes manifest and possibly untreatable. It relies on large numbers of apparently healthy people undergoing a system, run by non- (or para-)medical staff, who assess the environmental factors related to disease, and who, by using sophisticated equipment, can present the doctor with their assessment for him to practice his art, on a highly scientific basis. Such a system must have constant feed-back so that it evolves into an efficient preventative maintenance machine.

At present, the state of the art is in its infancy. There are still a great number of questions to be answered, and as medical technology advances, the efficiency of detection will improve. The figures given in this booklet are based on a sample of people from the senior management of British Industry. Their average age was in the late forties and ten per cent of them were more than twenty per cent overweight. Their mean income in 1972 was well over £5,000 per annum, and they were not, therefore, representative of the community as a whole, and it would be a pointless exercise trying to apply our system on a national basis. However, it is time that some kind of health maintenance was offered to people suffering from the stresses of modern life. This would have to be tailored to the needs of the community

and carried out under the supervision of our existing general practitioners. The emphasis in British health care must be shifted from the
'patching-up', sickness-orientated service to a comprehensive preventive service utilising all the modern techniques and machinery
that are available.

1.26

2
Heart Disease

H. Beric Wright, MB, FRCS

The Coronary Epidemic

Coronary heart disease is the biggest single killer of middle-aged men: between a third and a quarter of all men between thirty and sixty fail to reach retiring age because they die from this condition.

The death rate has gone up steadily since the war. It was just over 2,000 per million in 1951 and was nearly 3,500 in 1972—an alarming and significant increase in twenty years (Figure 2a). We believe that this toll of men in their prime, men who could and should go on making a significant contribution to the national prosperity, and of women who should not be prematurely widowed, can be reduced. This, we think, can be done in two ways: firstly, by a better understanding of the underlying processes of the disease; and secondly, by appropriate avoiding action backed up by regular maintenance.

This is what this series of booklets is all about and we hope that they will help people to live more sensibly—and longer.

What is Coronary Thrombosis?

The coronary arteries supply the muscle of the heart; they are the first vessels to arise from the aorta, just beyond the valves which control the blood flow round the body. These two relatively small but vital arteries run round the heart like a crown, hence their name.

Heart muscle, although it does have some special properties, is basically like all other body muscle, in that to function efficiently it needs, firstly, a good blood supply, and secondly, to be kept in training. Because of the anatomy of the coronary arteries, there is little overlap between their peripheral branches, so that should one, or a main branch get blocked, the muscle supplied is deprived of its blood supply.

Thrombosis means obstruction or blockage, thus coronary thrombosis means blockage of the coronary arteries. As a result of this blockage, the blood supply is halted and the area supplied is cut off from the source of supply. It is exactly the same situation as occurs when a power cable is cut or a main railway line blocked. There may

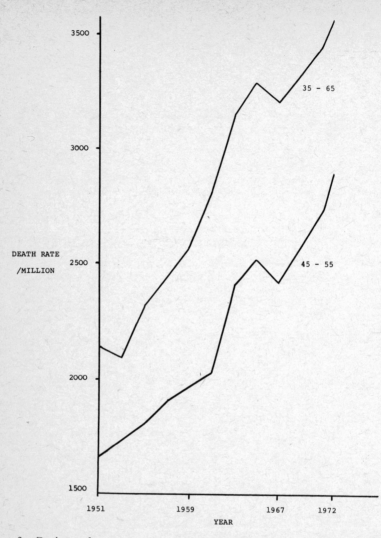

FIG 2a Death rates for men per million 1951–72. Upper line 35–65 age-group. Lower line 45–55 age-group.

In twenty years the death rate has increased from about 2,000 to 3,500 per million and in younger men from 1,600 to nearly 3,000. These figures demonstrate the 'epidemic' of coronary heart disease.

2.4

at a later date be other ways into the area, but essentially 'traffic' flow is stopped.

What happens to the heart depends on a number of factors, but obviously the extent of the blockage is the first and most important determinant. About a third of all coronary thromboses are fatal in the first few hours. If, however, the heart is robust enough to stand the shock and there is enough muscle left to continue the circulation, a good recovery can be expected. Even after severe thromboses, people—like Peter Sellers or Eric Morecambe, for instance—can live actively for years. Indeed, I believe that people can, if they learn their lesson, be even better or fitter than they were before. Thus, a serious coronary may be a sudden and unexpected disaster, a mild one can be both a warning and a blessing.

In any hydraulic system, flow can be stopped for three reasons: narrowing of the pipes, obstruction within the lumen or drop in circulatory pressure. Much the same is true of coronary heart disease. Athero- or arteriosclerosis is a generalised disease of the blood vessels which leads to their becoming both narrow and rigid. In addition, the internal lining becomes rough and ragged; this causes blood to clot, which clot or scab further narrows the vessel. Thus, narrowed vessels, or thickening of the arteries as it is called, reduces the blood flow to the part supplied. And this is as true of the heart as it is of the brain or legs. Unfortunately, although arteriosclerosis is a generalised disease of middle and older age, the coronary arteries tend to be sooner and separately involved; hence the sudden and unexpected deaths that this condition—now to be referred to as IHD—causes. IHD stands for ischaemic heart disease and ischaemia means reduced blood supply.

The mechanism which keeps the blood liquid during circulation and makes it clot when there is a leak in the system, i.e. after injury or rupture of a vessel, is extremely complex, but one of the factors is slowing down or stagnation. If blood stands still, as it were, it will clot. Obviously, if this happens in an artery or vein, the 'pipe' becomes blocked, blood cannot flow and the blockage tends to extend because of the further stagnation; thus a vicious circle is set up.

The two main factors then which cause a coronary thrombosis are disease of the artery wall and slowing of the blood flow. The factors which determine the seriousness of the event are the extent of the damage and the fitness of the heart to withstand the shock, i.e. flabby hearts survive less well than athletic ones, which means that the heart reflects, to a large degree, the health, fitness, etc. of its owner.

Causes of IHD

Sadly, and just to make it difficult, IHD is what we call multifactorial. By this, we mean that not one, but a variety of factors contribute to IHD. The situation is made more complicated by the fact that the various factors combine in different ways in different people and probably also, differently in the same person as he gets older. Most well-known diseases have a single or identifiable cause, like an allergy, or infection by a germ like the polio virus or typhoid bacillus. But in IHD any one or several of a number of factors contribute to coronary proneness—or as we are now inclined to say, 'risk'. We are increasingly using the term 'risk' because in an accountancy sense we can measure the risk, carry out a coronary audit and draw up a balance sheet.

There now follows a brief account of the various risk factors to help readers to identify them and, hopefully, to realise that—because many of them relate to the individual's personality and behaviour—salvation lies in living sensibly.

Genetic Predisposition

A coronary diathesis or tendency undoubtedly runs in families or is inherited. Just as some families are long-lived and survive IHD and other hazards, others live less long and die from one of a number of inherited diseases. Because IHD is multifactorial, the genetics of the situation are complicated, but to give one example, there is a familial genetically determined condition called familial hypercholesterolaemia. In this, babies are born with a high blood fat and will die very young unless this is detected and dealt with. Even then, however, the outlook is still gloomy.

The sons of coronary fathers and mothers—particularly the latter, in fact—are thus appreciably more likely to succumb to IHD than the siblings of long-lived parents. This does not mean that all the children will be affected but it does mean, in probability terms, that they are more likely to be affected.

What, the reader may ask, is the practical importance of this gloomy start to this booklet? There is nothing he can do about his inheritance . . . but there is, and this is why we mention it. The genetic situation provides the denominator to the equation: if this is good or low, greater risks can be taken with the other factors; if it is high, minor deviations of weight, smoking, blood pressure, etc. must be dealt with instantly.

Cholesterol, Fats and Lipids

We now know that the level of certain fats in the blood—the lipids— plays a major role in influencing both vessel wall disease and to a lesser extent blood clotting. If there is too much lipid in the blood, measured usually as cholesterol and triglyceride, this tends to get 'stuck' in the lining of the arteries and cause what we know as atherosclerosis.

Two main groups of factors seem to determine lipid levels. Obviously, the amount of fat in the diet is one, and the other, both less obvious and still only partially understood, is the way in which the body deals with or disposes of these lipids. And this is where the genetic factor plays a part. There is another complication in this part of the story, in that some kinds of lipids are more dangerous than others. Thus, what are chemically called saturated fats, play a far greater part in IHD than polyunsaturated fats. Roughly speaking these technical phrases mean animal fats and vegetable fats. One of the reasons advanced for the IHD epidemic is the greatly increased consumption of animal fats that goes with our higher standard of living. Clearly too, fat or obese people are likely to have a higher blood fat level than thin people.

Thus, the extent and type of fat consumed in the diet is one factor, the second is the way in which the individual metabolises the fat he takes. We now know that personality and genetic factors can influence all this and that stress, tension, anxiety and other hormonal conditions also play a part, which is why thin, tense, highly-strung people often have raised cholesterol and get coronaries.

The first step towards 'cholesterol control' is obviously to measure its level in the blood. This is relatively simple and at the same time, it is sensible to measure the other associated lipids, particularly the triglycerides. This should be done with the patient fasting, i.e. no breakfast etc., so that one is really measuring the basic level and not the effect of the last meal. All this is of vital importance because we know that individuals with raised lipids carry three to four times the coronary risk. Since obese people are more likely to have higher levels, the first step for such a person is to get their weight down to bogey and then review the situation. Should this not be sufficient, there is then a choice of either taking certain cholesterol lowering drugs or going on to a low cholesterol diet. Although this works well, it can be demanding and may well involve the whole family in altering their eating habits. Cholesterol comes in animal fats, dairy products, eggs and cheese, and therefore the diet consists of skim milk, lean meat, restricted eggs, vegetable oil for cooking, etc. In extreme cases an operation to short circuit part of the digestive system may be recommended.

In fact, lipid analysis has now become very sophisticated and four distinct types, each with their own characteristics and methods of treatment, have been differentiated. This can be very important because in the rather rare genetically determined cases, the very raised levels can and usually do lead to premature death at a tragically early age. A case was recently reported in the medical literature of a girl of seventeen having coronary thrombosis and raised blood pressure with fatal consequences. In the familial types of disease, it is usual to measure blood levels immediately after birth and start avoiding action straight away. At the Medical Centre recently, we were asked to carry out some blood tests on a seventeen-year-old girl who was generally unwell and off colour at school. Because we did our usual battery of tests, we found her cholesterol to be about three times what it should have been and she is now under long-term supervision.

Dramatic cases like these two are uncommon, but about a third of the people we see do have significant elevation of their lipids and evidence is now beginning to accrue which suggests that life expectancy is increased by dealing with it. Usually modest diet and attention to weight is all that is required. Diets are discussed in Booklet 3, and a weight table is included there.

Obesity

As weight control is dealt with in the third booklet in this series, little need be said about it here. Obesity is the commonest disease in developed countries and it is virtually always due to eating too much.

Thin people live longer than fat ones, partly because they have less to carry about, partly because their blood pressure is lower and partly perhaps because they tend to be more physically active (see also Booklet 3) and have lower lipid levels.

Professor John Yudkin and some others believe that increased consumption of sugar plays a major role in both obesity and IHD. The evidence for its specific 'toxic' effect is a bit thin, but as I said at the beginning of this section, thinness is a virtue and obesity is a lethal over-indulgence.

Exercise

There is now a lot of evidence to suggest that reasonable physical fitness protects against IHD. The classical investigation in this area showed that London Transport bus conductors, who run up and down stairs, had a lower coronary rate than the more sedentary drivers. Other and more detailed investigations have borne this out. In addition, the discipline—and discipline it is—for a middle-aged person to set out to take regular exercise, does produce other beneficial side effects. Fit people are stronger, more supple and more alert. Their hearts have a greater muscular reserve and work more effectively. Resting pulse rates are slower and recovery after exertion is more rapid.

Cigarette Smoking

Most of the propaganda against smoking, which is after all air pollution of a highly personalised kind, has been aimed at lung cancer. But this condition, which is far commoner in smokers, only kills about 1,060 per million per year compared with the 3,500 who die of IHD. But it is now quite clear that cigarette smokers, particularly heavy smokers, carry about three times the coronary risk. And as this risk is so real (remember one in three men die prematurely), this would seem to be both the best and an overwhelming reason for not smoking cigarettes.

Nicotine is a very subtle drug which has a complicated effect on the nervous system. It is a drug of addiction far commoner than alcohol or 'pot'. Roughly half the drug-addicts in this country are addicted to nicotine, and the evidence is that it does (through IHD, bronchitis and lung cancer) kill more people than the other two types of drug mentioned. Smoking is, of course, a good tranquilliser which is why people—particularly *cigarette* smokers—need to smoke to soothe their nerves. But it has other effects as well. Inhaling a cigarette puts up blood pressure—which can be harmful if the pressure is already high—and damages the lung tissue because of the direct irritant effect. Chronic bronchitis, known abroad as the 'English Disease', is caused by a mixture of environmental factors related to climate and living conditions, and inhalation. Smokers' cough should be regarded as a dangerous sign that the individual is damaging his lungs and certainly ought to stop. Non-coughers may be lucky and avoid bronchitis and possibly cancer, but they are still coronary candidates.

The most interesting effect of smoking, which has recently been discovered, is that it raises the carbon monoxide level in the blood. Before the advent of North Sea Gas—which contains largely methane—the coal gas oven was a favourite way of committing suicide. This was because carbon monoxide in high concentrations stops the blood transporting oxygen. In lower concentrations, of about fifteen per cent in heavy smokers, it lowers oxygen carrying efficiency, but more important, it seems to damage the walls of the smaller blood vessels. For chemical and hydraulic reasons, the carbon monoxide appears to concentrate on the outside of the blood column, thus exposing the vessel lining to the maximum concentration. The resulting damage may either predispose or encourage the other atherosclerotic processes already referred to.

Possibly a more important factor socially is the finding that non-smokers to some extent share this 'blood poisoning'. Non-smoking people in a smoky room have about a third the carbon monoxide level of smokers, as do those of us exposed to smog and traffic fumes. My colleague, Dr Alan Bailey, has been conducting some interesting Saturday morning experiments in his local pub. He has measured 'before and after' blood levels in smokers and non-smokers. The results (see Booklet 3) are rather frightening and should certainly stop people from inhaling cigarettes.

Stress, Personality and Behaviour

It is trite to say that everything that we do expresses our personality, but it is true. One can start assessing someone by their appearance, the clothes they wear, the tie they choose, the way they come into the

2.10

room, and so on. Similarly, whether or not one smokes, takes exercise, is overweight, is also a manifestation of personality. In general terms, over-indulgence or failure in these respects is a sign of fatalism, stupidity, lack of discipline, ignorance or weakness, etc.

But apart from this is the factor of stress and harassment. When we refer to someone as 'being stressed', we imply that life, or some part of it, has become too much for the individual and that he—or she—is showing signs of wear. As stress is so important in our adjustment to life, it is perhaps worth more detailed analysis. Indeed, understanding stress and knowing oneself in relation to it, is the key to survival—from coronary thrombosis and other diseases.

Stress is a term which has come to be misunderstood in the process of popularisation. Strictly speaking, it comes from engineering where it implies an ability to withstand strain. Thus, an engineer can design a bridge, or an architect a building, to withstand a designated amount of strain. The strength of the materials used is both predictable and measurable. Should he get his sums wrong, the building will blow down in a gale, as can happen with roofs and cooling towers; or, if the material alters, as with some concrete recently used, it gets weaker and collapses. Similarly, if too heavy a vehicle goes over a bridge the girders will bend.

The construction industry has taken this further by, for instance, increasing the strength of concrete by pre-stressing it. The same can, in fact, occur in individuals by conditioning, training and experience. The whole basis, for instance, of military training and discipline is to condition the troops against the normal panic of battle stress.

Biologically, all living things are in conflict both with their environment and with each other. Plants compete for space and nutrition and have to live with the climate or perish. Over many generations various species learn to survive under certain conditions, the successful ones become cleverer at this and pass their characteristics on to their young—which is, of course, the basis of evolution.

Humans, being biological entities, can be expected to behave in exactly the same way and indeed they do, although their reactions are much more complicated. What all living things need, to keep them 'vital', is challenge. Plants, animals and humans need to be challenged by the environment, firstly to 'keep them on their toes', and secondly, particularly for humans, to give them the satisfaction of succeeding.

As far as man is concerned, he had, at least until recently, learned to control the environment and most of his 'challenge' comes from the psycho-social, rather than the physical environment. Obviously, parts of the third world are still challenged by the need for food and warmth and in other places various sorts of pollution are currently presenting environmental problems.

If challenge is a biological necessity, which it is in practice, it is to be expected that there will be a biologically acceptable defence mechanism against too much challenge—and this is what stress is all about. Challenge in its various forms presents the strain which engineering expects and 'stress' is what happens when life becomes too much for us. We opt out of the challenging situation by becoming 'stressed'.

Medically and technically we know a great deal about certain diseases, particularly those with an identifiable cause like tuberculosis or poliomyelitis, but even with regard to them, it is far from clear what determines why one individual gets infected—in say an epidemic—and why another will survive. When it comes to more generalised conditions like depression, indigestion, asthma and psoriasis, etc. we really know very little about the infective agent.

I believe, and by no means would all doctors agree with this, that most illness or 'dis-ease' arises from the individual's need to opt out of a stressful situation, i.e. disease is biologically a defence mechanism to get someone off the hook of too much challenge. It is also a fact of experience that happy, well-adjusted people who have a capacity for enjoyment, are seldom ill. But miserable people who are continually worried or grumbling about how hard life is—you can often hear the chips rattling on their shoulders—tend to be riddled with aches and pains: they really are dis-eased. It is also worth noting in this respect that, again biologically, pain is a call for help. When we experience pain we are discomforted and we ask for social sympathy from family and friends and technical sympathy from the healing professions.

The difficulty of making this relatively simple hypothesis credible lies in the fact that the great majority of our reactions are subconscious rather than conscious, so that the chain of cause and effect, in behavioural terms, is drowned in subconscious or learned responses which are exhibited either as symptoms or behavioural disturbances. Thus, left to ourselves, we have no idea why we become ill or why we get asthma, migraine, skin spots, irritability, insomnia or depression. In practice, this is not entirely true because most people realise that they do not sleep when they are worried, or that severe anxiety tends to stop them thinking straight on other issues.

Space does not permit me to go into this in more detail, but two illustrations might help in the general understanding of the philosophy. Many years ago, a psychiatric colleague of mine was asked to see a fifteen-year-old girl who had asthma so badly that its control required large doses of steroids undesirable in a child this age. The story he elicited was as follows.

The girl was bright and had done well at school and got a grammar school place. She had an extremely ambitious mother who was pushing her. This involved insisting on the grammar school, whereas the girl wanted to go to the secondary modern with her class-mates. By developing asthma, she—entirely subconsciously—not only got out of school, but kept her mother away from work to look after her. Once all this had been pointed out, the situation could be discussed rationally.

Some time ago I saw a rather pathetic middle-aged man, who walked into my consulting room and launched into a long account of his (severe) indigestion. This dated from the death of his mother about twenty years previously. My spontaneous response was 'Good God, haven't you got over that yet?' He had traded on this sympathy, through two marriages, for twenty years and I was not popular for pulling his prop away so suddenly.

Against this background, it is worth pointing out that it is conflict—perceived and unperceived—which is so stressful and which produces defensive symptoms. Unsolved problems cause conflict and once the individual realises where the conflict lies, he or she can begin to see the answer, even if this is to accept that there is no immediate solution. 'Live with it and stop worrying' may be the only way out. Similarly, if someone has stress symptoms related to situations—like the man who always vomited when he went to see his dominating father—the fact that the cause can be identified makes the situation easier. Many such symptoms can, when so recognised, be regarded as a friendly warning that margins of (behavioural) tolerance are being approached.

Having said all this, it must be noted that not all dis-ease can be dealt with so easily and individuals do have widely differing threshholds of tolerance. An anxious inadequate person will break down under very modest stress, while a tougher one will be seen to survive intolerable conditions. Similarly, people's thresholds vary between work and home or intellectual and executive activities. Thus, the good technocrat may be outstanding in his laboratory and hopeless at management of people, or I may get on with one boss whom you would find totally incompatible. The stress situation is both highly personal and strictly related to time and event. We have called this the personality–environment equation. If it is in balance all will be well. If not, there are likely to be stress and defence symptoms.

This is, of course, a gross over-simplification of a very complicated series of interrelated situations, which arise from the personality and the environment. No-one is indestructable and we all have a breaking point. When life becomes too much for us—we 'get stressed', something goes wrong with our reactions and we develop aberrant behaviour or get symptoms of dis-ease. These can take any form, from an acute anxiety state to insomnia and irritability, to indigestion, muscle or tension pain, migraine or spots. The stressed person resorts to pain, illness or discomfort, to get him—in biological terms—off the stress hook. He opts out of this bit of the rat race to recharge his batteries and recover for the next round.

Personality obviously plays a large part in this. Placid people get less excited by conflicts than do highly-strung ones. Extroverts tend to react better to many social situations than do introverts and so on. From this, it should be clear that, in very simple terms, there is little doubt that highly strung, nervous or anxious people, take much more out of themselves than do others. Similarly, worriers get more frayed than non-worriers.

Another factor here is inherent ability; stress is related to morale and there is nothing like success and achievement to keep morale high and this mitigates against being stressed. And being stressed is not the same as (successfully) carrying a lot of responsibility or holding down a demanding job. It is the person who fails to do this, rather than the one who succeeds, who exhibits stress. Thus one would expect to and on the whole one does find more stress below the top—in middle management—than in the leaders. In order to succeed they have to be able to deal with the situation.

This does, however, need qualifying by making the point that people are vulnerable to stress on several fronts; thus the man who is good at his job may be dreadful at home. Domestic stress is just as prevalent as work stress, and anxiety from family troubles, teenage children and so on, can destroy people or drive them to drink, just as much as the collapse of the Stock Exchange or a bloody-minded boss.

What all this does, is to make the stressed person much more coronary prone in a variety of ways. He may smoke more, drink more, get over-tired, fail to take his holidays, over-eat for comfort and so on. Another point to realise in this area, is that fatigue, although quite different from stress, is obviously related. The tired person will be prone to all sorts of hazards and in addition his stress threshold will be lowered by his fatigue. Anxiety from whatever cause is also very tiring, so that the ability to tolerate anxiety is again a major factor in dealing with stress.

Alcohol

Although not directly concerned as a coronary risk factor, over-indulgence in alcohol is closely related. Management life is full of temptations to drink too much and a fairly strict discipline is required not to get on to a slippery slope of regular heavy consumption of more than four or five drinks a day. Moderate drinking (up to four drinks a day) can be a good release, a helpful end-of-day relaxer and useful social lubricant—more than this can destroy performance, reputation and the liver, which is the organ mainly concerned with dealing with, or metabolising alcohol. In addition, alcohol is a high calorie food and if taken in conjunction with too much bread, potatoes, and sweets, can lead to obesity.

We have, for the last year or so, been doing a special liver test which shows up early and rapidly reversible damage due to alcohol. We are concerned about the number of people over fifty who show such damage. They are by no means alcoholics, but they are drinking more than they can deal with.

It is easy to see how the stressed, tired, anxious man who has a lot of problems round his neck, or the travelling business man, lonely in hotels or being entertained too much, can easily become 'weakened' by mild over-indulgence. This may make him smoke more

2.15

and generally neglect his physical state. (He is also likely to be over-weight.)

Like everything else but cigarettes, alcohol in moderation—or even the odd binge—is splendid, but taken too much, too regularly, it becomes part of the coronary picture, a looser of driving licences and a cause of domestic distress.

Miscellaneous Factors

Hormones

No-one quite knows why the incidence of IHD is less in women than men and at an appreciably later age. This seems to be related to the different hormone balance in women and the fact that on the whole, women do not get IHD until at least ten years after the change of life. At this time, there is an alteration of hormone output and a disappearance of oestrogen, the main female hormone. It would seem that oestrogen has some protective effect on the cardiovascular system. Similarly, although there have been fewer case studies, eunuchs and castrati are believed not to get coronaries. Unfortunately large doses of oestrogen, which are used to treat cancer of the prostate, causes a biochemical castration, so that this line of treatment has little use. It is clear, however, that the steroid hormone system does play a part and this may be one of the mechanisms whereby stress is involved. In any case, many of the body systems are co-ordinated by hormones.

Hard Water

Recent very detailed statistical work has shown that people who live in hard water areas have a lower rate of IHD than those in soft. There are reasonable biochemical reasons for this, related to the chemistry of arterial hardening, which is part of arterio sclerosis. It could thus be wise not to go out of one's way to drink artifically softened water.

Other Diseases

We have already mentioned familial hypercholesterolaemia as a cause of IHD. There are a number of other conditions which may contribute indirectly. The commonest of these is probably gout, which, if uncontrolled, damages the kidney. Almost any kidney damage puts up blood pressure which then affects the heart. Gout is a relatively easy condition to control, as the regular consumption of one or two drugs keeps the uric acid in the blood below danger level.

The Coronary Audit and Health Maintenance

Before he can certify a balance sheet or set of accounts, an auditor has to go through the books and see that the figures are correct. In advising an individual about his health, particularly with regard to coronary risk factors, we try to do much the same. We take certain measurements, assess the individual in relation to his personality and way of life and then try and draw up a balance sheet. Having done this, in relation to a detailed health check, we can then advise him accordingly. Thus, low-risk, or fit people, can be reassured, medium-risk can be advised about altering their way of life and high-risk people are usually sent for a specialist opinion and possibly more active treatment. All this has the advantage of giving the patient a rational basis for the advice he is given because it can be explained to him.

Going back to the coronary risk factors, we need, on the physical side, to know the following things:

1. Age
2. Height and weight, to calculate relative weight—i.e. is he fat or thin, and by how much?
3. Lung function—has his lung tissue and respiratory reserve been destroyed by disease or filter tips?
4. Blood pressure and cardiograph (see section below)
5. Chest and other X-rays
6. Hearing and vision
7. Urine test for diseases like diabetes and kidney upset
8. Blood count for anaemia, etc.
9. Blood biochemical profile with particular attention to lipids and liver function
10. Clinical examination
11. Personality-environment assessment and life-style audit.

2.17

In my view the last item is the critical one, because it forms the basis of the advice one can give the individual. He needs to be looked at under the headings of work, home and leisure, as well as being assessed on his family history and personal habits, like drinking, smoking, exercise, holidays, commuter travel, work travel in this country and abroad, etc. The examining doctor should, in our view, be interested in and knowledgeable about the businessman's life. Hopefully, too, the man will come as part of an executive group who will all be seen by the same doctor. The doctor thus knows and understands the company and develops some insight into the pressures and personalities that dominate it.

Having done all this and got the relevant facts, the doctor can then make up his mind, firstly, whether the man is at risk and, secondly, if he is, the extent of this risk and what avoiding action is appropriate. It is often said that all we do at the Medical Centre is to tell people that they are too fat, smoke too much and ought to get off their backsides. But although we need to do this in relation to the coronary risk factors already listed, we are also rather better able, because of the background, to push people into, for instance, stopping smoking. Obviously too, we have to be careful that the treatment is not worse than the disease. If a man is currently under tremendous pressure, it is silly to choose that moment to make him go through the tortures of stopping smoking. But if at the same time his cardiograph is disturbed and his blood pressure raised, one must take the risk if he is to have the best chances of survival. One can legitimately threaten him, his wife and the company, with potential death and let them or him take the decision.

I personally take the view, but not all my colleagues would agree with me, that on the whole, people both have a right and ought to know what is wrong with them. If they do not like or are worried by the answer, this is their worry, but the motivation to change is likely to be good. Thus, we tend to tell people what is wrong with them.

This approach can perhaps be illustrated with two examples. Many years ago, I saw a silly, over-indulgent, youngish man, for about the third time. Since his last visit, he had started cigarette smoking again and his cardiograph showed distinct changes. I showed him the before and after tracings and said that he must stop smoking or the situation would deteriorate. His cardiograph went back to normal, but al-

2.18

though I have not seen him much since, I have reason to believe that he has grown a new set of less lethal vices.

Secondly, take myself. Both my parents are alive, well into their eighties. I do not smoke cigarettes and as a family 'thing' have low blood pressure. I am about ten per cent overweight, but reckon that in the light of the other findings this is acceptable. If, on the other hand, I had a patient whose mother died of a coronary at the age of fifty-five—a rare event—who smoked cigarettes, had mildly raised blood pressure and was similarly overweight, he would have to take action.

This is the principle of the coronary risk audit and as backing for the way in which doctors ought to advise people, it works reasonably well. Dr. Bailey has used his computer to identify coronary risk patients coming to our Medical Centre. (See figures 2b and 2c.). He has then rated them in a numerical scale, by allocating points, in a rather arbitrary way, to the various factors. What is so frightening about this exercise is that rather few people get really good marks, most are borderline and again few are really bad—they have already died.

Health Maintenance Surveillance

We believe that preventive maintenance on people is just as relevant as it is for motor cars, or plant and machinery. You do not wait until your car breaks down to have it serviced, nor do you wait for toothache before going to the dentist—you go regularly to protect against such eventualities.

You, the reader, as an individual, do not know what your blood pressure is, what your cardiograph looks like, or what your blood lipids are, unless they have all been measured. It is only by regularly assessing coronary risk factors that one can begin to identify high-risk people and do something about them.

For these and many other reasons, we believe most strongly that if the toll of IHD is to be halted, people must have regular health maintenance. By constructing a log-book, with annual or biannual

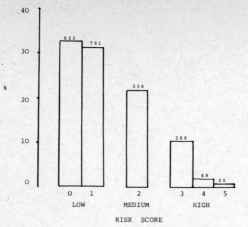

FIG 2b   A random sample of well over 2000 men aged 30–50 were rather arbitarily scored on a six-point scale for three coronary risk factors, viz. cholesterol, smoking, blood pressure.

The scores are shown in this figure. About 65% of the group can be regarded as low risk, 20% medium risk and 15% high risk.

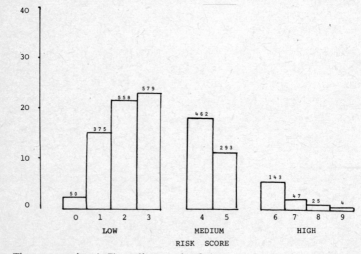

FIG 2c   The same sample as in Figure 2b was reclassified on a ten-point scale with additional risk factors, viz. family history, obesity, exercise.

The scores for all six risk factors are given here. Those scoring three or less (about 60% of the group) rate as low risk, 30% rate as medium risk and about 10% as high risk.

The scoring is rather arbitrary but the figures do demonstrate the high proportion of 'well men' with a significantly high risk.

2.20

insertions, one can easily monitor the situation. The initial examination charts the baseline and subsequent ones will instantly recognize improvement or deterioration from this. The other day, we had a man who had been coming to us for several years. His cholesterol had always been a bit high and slowly climbing. Quite suddenly at his last visit, it was found to have shot up even higher, which finding rang all the alarm signals and the 'life boat' was called out.

It is also worth noting that although we cannot and do not guarantee survival, continued normal findings can be regarded as reasonably reassuring. In the present state of the art, a few seemingly normal people will get coronaries and a few bad ones may survive. But, by and large, risk factor rating is a good statistical help to giving individuals the best advice.

Blood Pressure and the Cardiograph

The heart is a pump and the blood vessels are the circulation system— very like a central heating system in a house or block of flats. In ordinary hydraulics, should the calibre of the pipes be reduced, the circulatory pressure required to maintain the flow must be increased pro rata. But similarly, the more work that the pump has to do, the sooner it is likely to wear out; and the higher the circulatory pressure, the greater the chance of leaks. Exactly the same is true of the human circulatory system. We do not know which comes first, higher blood pressure or reduced vessel calibre (arteries exposed to increased pressure react by losing their elasticity), but we do know that hypertension (raised blood pressure) does predispose to several dangerous sequelae like heart failure, strokes and coronary ischaemia.

The person with hypertension, which often goes with obesity and kidney disease, is more prone to IHD in its various forms and has a considerably reduced life expectancy for several reasons.

The heart has a fairly complicated internal communications system which co-ordinates the rate and rhythm of each beat. The signal for this to happen spreads 'electrically' through the communication system, in a constant pattern. By taking a sensitive tracing of the propagation of this electrical impulse one can learn a great deal about the heart and its conduction system. Such a tracing is called an electro-cardiograph (ECG) and is done quickly and easily by placing electrodes on the skin over the heart and on the limbs. It is a guide as

2.21

to the state of the muscle and its blood supply. Early changes can often be picked up and sometimes reversed. It is also extremely useful to have a baseline tracing, taken early in middle age, from which subsequent minor change can be noted. When someone has a significant coronary thrombosis with destruction of a lot of muscle, this will obviously be reflected in the ECG as, to a degree, will be the recovery. Most coronaries, however, leave a permanent ECG abnormality.

Avoiding Action

It is very difficult to be dogmatic about the interrelationships and responsibilities of the individual and the organisation for which he works. One can say that individuals should look after their own health. Equally companies ought not to destroy people by being over-demanding or unreasonable. By the same token, it may well be sound economics for the company to pay some attention to looking after its staff, at least as well as it does its machinery. I believe that this complicated relationship is best looked at as a marriage in which both parties have responsibilities and duties, which lead to them both getting enough out of the deal to make it worthwhile and productive.

To give a simple, if still neglected example, many managers have to do a lot of business travel and this can be extremely tiring, especially if it is against time. Flying east or west interferes with the biological time clock called circadian rhythm. The body gets used to a UK time base; suddenly taking it to America and turning night into day is asking too much of it—very like expecting members of Parliament to be intelligent at three in the morning when they ought normally to be asleep. For this and other related reasons, sensible companies lay down travel rules which minimise the demand on the traveller. Thus, it is essential to have at least one good long night on the east and two nights and a day on the west coast of America, before starting work. Equally, the same or longer pauses must be insisted on when the traveller returns. It is difficult, particularly for the more junior staff member to demand this for himself; he must be 'given it' by the rules. Travel stress is a major cause of executive strain and it is discussed in detail in Chapter 8 of *Executive Ease and Dis-Ease* (H. Beric Wright, Gower Press, Epping).

Although the borderline between individual and company responsibility is blurred and overlaps, it is perhaps worth looking at the main areas under the two headings, even at the expense of some repetition.

Action by the Individual

The most important single item in the individual's survival kit is what we call insight. The more one can look at oneself objectively in relation to the stresses, challenges and conflict of life—and know what it might do to you—the less likelihood there is of disaster.

Stress, in its damaging form, is, as we have briefly said, related to personality–environment imbalance. Thus knowing something about your own limitations and what the danger signs from being overstretched are, can be of the greatest help in surviving. Another factor here is the ability to equate, reasonably accurately, aspirations and attributes, i.e. it is the over-ambitious man who tries to go further or be better than he in fact is, who comes unstuck.

Early in life, it is obviously sensible to aim, if not at the stars, at least at the horizon, and to strive hard to establish a good niche in life. But around middle age it is sensible to do a stock check and realise that life is for living, which may involve settling for what you have got and getting fun out of other things. Indeed, one of the keys to dealing with stress is to be a balanced man. We all like to think that we can chop ourselves up into slices and then take one bit to work and leave the rest at home. But, of course, this does not work. Domestic anxiety, or even a sleepless night from an ailing child, feeds into the work situation just as much as does an incompatible boss, redundancy or anxiety over a strike.

The converse is equally true, however, in that pleasure, satisfaction and success obtained outside work, help to balance the stresses of work. Thus, the man who won a prize for his model aeroplane or at the rose show, goes to the office with a lighter step than the man who worked at his papers or the doctor who sat writing articles rather than gardening! For this type of reason, it is absolutely essential that businessmen, after the age of forty-five, go out of their way to remain human and develop outside interests and contacts. The work-centred man is both vulnerable and boring—and if you do not believe me, ask his family.

Obviously, there are a lot of relatively simple things a sensible man will build into his life style. They might be outlined as follows:

Diet and Weight

If you are one of those lucky people, who can eat as much as they like of everything; bully for you. Most of us, however, are good converters and have to watch our calorie intake. Loading in more calories than we need merely leads to them being banked as fat. Income must equal expenditure and the ways of doing this are described in Booklet 3. I always look at this in terms of eating the things I enjoy, because food and drink are a major pleasure and, leaving out the rest, I would rather have my calories in gin and peanuts than in bread and potatoes and this is the way to permit it. There is no place for sugar in tea or coffee, or biscuits in the morning if you have a weight problem. Should there be a cholesterol problem, a low fat diet will be essential and the whole family must co-operate.

Exercise

Keeping reasonably physically fit has advantages over and above the need to protect the heart from a coronary risk. The fit man is likely to be more alert and resilient, less tired and better balanced. Middle-aged people ought to do a regular exercise schedule like the Canadian 5BX. Also they ought to get out of doors at the week-end, walk up stairs and round the office. Action is an attitude of mind and sloth is a sin. All this again is looked at in detail in Booklet 3. Taking the dog out for a reasonably long walk before going to bed is another good discipline.

Smoking

Pipes and cigars in moderation and not inhaled are allowed. Cigarettes should be avoided at all costs. Stopping smoking is, for most addicts, extremely difficult. It is an addiction and stopping produces all the acute withdrawal symptoms that go with other forms of addiction; if not 'Pink Elephants', at least irritability, paranoia and bloody-mindedness. Great toleration is required from family and friends, but it is worth it.

One of the things that nicotine does is to liberate adrenalin, which in turn liberates glucose from the liver. Thus every cigarette gives a shot of glucose—hence the craving for sweets and sweet things that most people get when they try to stop. This may well, and often does, lead to a mild increase in weight. But it is better to deal with the smoking first and when this has stabilised, to deal with the weight as a secondary problem. Obviously, too, it is legitimate to choose the right time to stop: annual budget, end of financial year, union agreements, etc. are clearly trying enough without this additional burden. It is also worth noting that the children of non-smokers are far less likely to smoke than those whose parents do.

Drink

In the end, this must be a personal decision, but the exposed individual (and businessmen are exposed in a variety of ways) must watch his alcohol consumption. It is a good exercise periodically to demonstrate that it can be done without, either during the week or at the week-end. Lunch-time drinking is another difficult area, because there is no doubt that an alcoholic lunch detracts from the afternoon performance. Similarly, it is less than fair on one's wife regularly to come home late smelling of drink and not wanting to have one with her.

Outside Interests

As has been implied, these are essential as middle age advances, not only do they give balance to the stress situation, but they also make the individual a more useful citizen by broadening his judgement. It does not much matter what the 'interests' are, provided they satisfy the individual. Some should involve physical activity, preferably with the family, and in my view others might well entail ploughing something back into the community through social involvement. Inevitably, as they get more senior, professional people tend to get sucked into trade and professional associations. Personally, I am always a bit suspicious of these, prestigious though they may be. They are mostly a bit too close to work and tend to involve the same people and also they tend to entail boring dinners and endless committee meetings. But anything is better than nothing.

2.25

Sleep, Holidays and Fatigue

I am always very suspicious of the man who is too busy to take his holiday and works too long hours. He usually has a disease called delusions of indispensability and should be shooed away into the sun. The busier one is, the more important it is, except in dire crisis, to get proper holidays.

Sleep too, is precious, some people are lucky and can sleep anywhere and at any time, others find it much more difficult and have to go out of their way to cultivate sleep. I am a believer in the judicious use of sleeping pills, particularly in relation to travel.

Trying not to run down by getting over-tired, is a major part of the 'know yourself' kit. It is worth realising how inefficient one becomes when thoroughly worn out, and for a variety of reasons in this state, the individual is much more coronary prone. It is better to let up and make someone else do the work, than to blow a gasket.

Family Life

There is not space in this booklet to do more than mention the importance and the frequent failure of business marriage. By failure, I do not necessarily mean the divorce rate, but I do mean the rather low quality of the relationship between the couple. Wives of very involved people tend to get left with house, home and children, and father tends not to pull his weight with the latter and has no relationship with them should there be an adolescent crisis.

I believe that wives should drive a much harder bargain in getting higher priority attention out of their husbands. Also, of course, they have a vested interest in not becoming one of the thirty per cent of business widows. Thus, they can strive to keep their man alive by stopping him getting exhausted, insisting on leisure and exercise and co-operating with his diet so that he is sensibly and not over fed. Women, to a degree, try to justify their role by demonstrating their culinary competence. This is all very well, but Dad did have lunch at the office and would benefit from a light supper. More is said about this in Booklet 3.

In a very small number of cases an ambitious wife can drive her husband to a coronary by expecting and demanding too much from him. Beware of this.

2.26

The Role of the Company

The concept of the company is rather amorphous and hard to identify precisely. Although in the ultimate, companies are made up of teams of people and those at the top do have very considerable power, organisations do also have an on-going personality based on their traditional behaviour. Often this can be a menace because it can be very frustrating for keen youngsters to be stuck into a rather fuddy-duddy mould and made to conform.

Basically, those at the top of an organisation have a responsibility to create an environment in which people can flourish. If they get this right, the firm will too. If it is badly wrong, the coronary rate will be high, because the staff will be over-stressed and harassed. There are always 'horses for courses', and no individual is universally compatible or omnipotential. Management and individuals must co-operate to slot people into the right holes, monitor the environment to see that the challenges are right, and see that there are end-products to people's activities. It is also desirable to ventilate grievances, discuss frustrations and tell staff how they are doing.

If a man is showing signs of strain, the reasons should be sought and some of the burden shifted. Willing horses should not be slaughtered and executives made to share and delegate. Proper working habits and procedures should be enforced. This can include holidays, days off, travel rules, decent offices, supervised canteen menus, control of drinking and so on. Travel rules have already been discussed and are a major way in which the organisation can protect the individual. If at all possible, long distance travel should, in my view, be first class. It should also be emphasised that entertainment is work and that travellers are not expected to work a longer week than they would at home.

Executive Health Examinations

From what has been said, regular health maintenance examinations are the cornerstone of 'avoiding a coronary'. No-one knows what their vital statistics are, unless they are regularly measured and monitored. We now call this presymptomatic diagnosis, because most of the early signs which lead to becoming a high coronary risk case, cause few noticeable changes until it is too late. We cannot yet prove statistically the benefits of early treatment—largely because the statistical method and the length of follow-up make the experiment difficult and expensive.

Another difficulty arises from the multifactorial nature of the condition. By stopping smoking, more than just this one factor is altered, including the individual's attitude to life and work. Incidentally, it is worth noting that as far as IHD is concerned, the benefits of stopping have recently been measured and delineated, from Framingham in America. But by and large, anyone, particularly anyone under fifty, is well-advised to take preventive action if found to be in a high risk category. This may even involve stepping sideways or seriously considering a change of job to get out of an intolerable or uncongenial situation. This may be a counsel of perfection at present, but many people are happier to become bigger fish in smaller ponds— even at a reduced income.

At the Medical Centre, we run health schemes for over five hundred companies, so we can claim both expertise and that this is a facility that more and more organisations provide for their staff. In addition, a growing number of self-employed people are coming because they realise how important their health is. Usually, the company pays for the examination and may or may not want a detailed report about the findings. We like the report facility (with the consent and knowledge of the individual) because it allows us to deal with or discuss medical findings which arise from, or influence the work situation. The pros and cons of all this are discussed in a booklet available at the Centre.

Another related and much appreciated facility is the provision, by the company, of sickness insurance either through BUPA or a similar policy. With this cover, both know that any medical situation can be rapidly and effectively dealt with, without financial anxiety.

If the medical is carried out by skilled and experienced doctors, it provides an annual forum where personal and other problems can be discussed and the risk factors calmly and objectively assessed. Unless done in this way and in relation to a previously charted base line, the examination has little more value than the average, rather badly done life insurance examination.

2.28

Dealing with Company Problems

The one or two people at the top of any organisation of any size whatever, have a responsibility, either directly or through a designated nominee, to keep up an over-view on what the company is doing to its staff and vice versa. Often in my view, the people in the company are reluctant to be cruel to be kind. Passengers are carried too long, instead of being put out, or back, to find their correct level, and problem children are not dealt with.

The most extraordinary thing about alcoholics is the way in which they are tolerated—almost being kept as pets, by workmates and family. Everyone knows that 'old George' drinks far too much, but no-one will seriously help him to stop. Recently, I saw a man who finally had to resign his partnership because he was ineffectual. He had been sent on two cruises 'to get over it', but no-one thought of treating his depression. Anyone who begins to fall down on the job, particularly after a previously good performance, should be reviewed and, if necessary, 'medicaled': there is nearly always a reason—which may originate domestically rather than at work. But unless the reason is found, the situation is unlikely to be properly resolved.

Alcoholics, who exist every now and again in all organisations, are their own worst enemy. Because of the personality disturbance, they really have to be confronted with their disease, in order to deal with it. Often what the Americans have called 'job jeopardy' is by far the best weapon. Management must have the man in and say 'unless . . . '. And they must mean it. Not only must the individual be helped, but the others must see that although sympathetic handling is available, passengers are not carried.

Conclusion

Coronary thrombosis is a contemporary epidemic which has so far defied treatment. This is, firstly, because it is multifactorial in origin, unlike diseases like typhoid and tuberculosis, and, secondly, because much of the damage may have been done before the sufferer is aware of it. Thus, the man who gets dyspepsia or a duodenal ulcer may be luckier than the one who gets a coronary. The former rings much earlier symptomatic bells which demand treatment.

But the early signs of coronary thrombosis can often be detected by presymptomatic diagnosis (screening) and if suitably analysed they can be treated. Many of them are behavioural in origin and can be mitigated by the individual himself. First, he has to understand himself in relation to the pressures, second, he has to accept certain disciplines about weight, smoking, exercise, holidays, travel, etc. and third, he may have to realise that he was not quite the guy he thought he was. He has, in middle age, to re-equate his aspirations and his attributes and realise that life is for living. 'Stop trying too hard and accept a more modest role in life', could be a life saving motto for the middle-aged. Most of us are 'Mr Average' and we cannot all be generals and field-marshals. Social or hierarchial status is not the only satisfaction in life. Challenge is essential: failure can be disastrous.

3
Fitness Without Fantasies

Alan Bailey, MB, MRCP
H. Beric Wright, MB, FRCS
Harry N. Levitt, OBE, FRCGP

Introduction

At first sight it might seem unusual to consider the effects of smoking, taking exercise and obesity in the same booklet. But the subjects have much in common. Two of the simplest tests available to doctors to detect illness are measurement of the pulse rate and the blood pressure. The pulse tells how fast the heart is working and what state the blood vessels are in; the blood pressure tells how forceful the heart is; both are measurements of how hard the heart is working.

Cigarette smoking, taking exercise and being overweight, all increase the work done by the heart—manifesting itself by a rise in pulse rate and blood pressure. Yet the exercise is healthy but the other two factors are not. All are interdependent, linked by physiological and psychological pathways which are discussed in this booklet. Cigarette smoking and average weight have increased dramatically in this country in this century, and the amount of exercise taken has declined similarly. In their different ways they cause breathlessness, and are the subject of numerous documentaries and statements in Britain today. Much research is carried out on the effects of smoking, sedentary life and obesity on the human body, in an attempt to understand the nature of the diseases with which they are associated (either beneficially or detrimentally) and this booklet attempts to unravel the facts from the theories and concludes with a practical approach to an exciting problem.

Tobacco

Tobacco in cigar form has been with us for nearly 400 years. The Spanish introduced cigars to Britain around 1600, returning from expeditions to the New World. The cigar was a symbol of wealth, whereas the paper-wrapped cigarette was the invention of beggars, who used tobacco from discarded cigar butts. However, by the late nineteenth century, machines were producing cigarettes in increasing quantities to satisfy a popular demand, mainly among men, for the effects of smoking. Tobacco usage in Britain since 1900 has steadily increased and since the 1930s women have shown a similar trend (see Figure 3a).

The tobacco plant is now grown mainly in Africa and the Americas and treated in a number of ways to produce the varieties of cigarettes on the market today. In Britain the most popular tobacco is 'flue-cured' from Virginia. When the tobacco is ignited it produces a number of substances. Among the most important are nicotine, a strong drug (although produced in very small quantities by one cigarette), a combination of tars and the gas

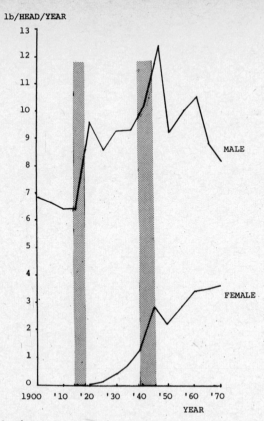

FIG 3a   Trends in tobacco consumption this century. The male graph includes cigar and pipe smokers but the female only cigarettes. The falling off in consumption per head in the last twenty years for men is largely due to the change to filter tipped cigarettes. Hatched areas show the war years which have a marked influence on tobacco consumption. (Tobacco Research Council, 1972)

carbon monoxide. The popularity of cigarette smoking is due partly to its social effects, and partly to the effect of nicotine on the body. The social side of smoking includes the breaking of the ice in difficult situations, the pleasure of the ritual, offering around, lighting, sucking and having something to do with the hands. Smokers are socially acceptable to each other; it provides a kind of bond, although less so to the non-smoker. The pleasant physiological effects are largely due to the action of the nicotine on the brain and other organs, producing a mild feeling of well-being and relaxation. Smoking is habit-forming and usually addictive—the difference

3.4

being that the addict forms a physical and mental dependence on it and suffers ill-effects (withdrawal symptoms) when he attempts to stop. Such symptoms in smokers are usually mild—one of the most persistent being a constant craving. The dangerous effects of cigarette smoking may be divided into the short-term and the long-term dangers.

The Dangers of Smoking

Smoking may produce immediate poisonous effects such as vomiting, headaches and disturbances of vision. Single or frequent cigarettes may produce inflammation of the sinuses (sinusitis), the throat and wind pipe and they represent a fire hazard particularly for elderly or invalid people. They produce a blunting of the sense of smell, making the smoker unaware that he himself and his clothes often smell of stale cigarettes. Taste is also usually blunted by constant smoking.

The long-term effects are more devastating, leading ultimately to either chronic disability or death. To understand fully the long-term hazards, it is necessary to look more closely at the physiological effects of smoking. The internal lining of the windpipe and the larger of the air ducts into the lungs consist of a smooth layer of tiny cells forming what is called a membrane. This membrane is moist and has tiny hairs standing up from it which have a continual sweeping-type movement, rather like corn moving in a gentle wind. The air we breathe is full of tiny particles, often too small to see, which could be damaging to the lungs if they were not trapped by the hairs, wafted out again or absorbed by the cleansing fluid of the membrane. When a large quantity of fluid has to be produced to combat the dirty outside world we call it phlegm, and assist its outward movement by coughing. The first noticeable action of tobacco smoke inhaled into the lungs is to paralyse the protective action of this hairy lining and cause an increase in the normal fluid production to compensate. Continual exposure eventually leads the hairs to be permanently damaged, the membrane to thicken (in order to provide more fluid) and the fluid to become so excessive that it forms thick phlegm. This is the beginning of the smokers cough, and explains why smokers are far more susceptible to chest disorders than are non-smokers, the protective mechanism against germs having been largely paralysed.

Thickening and inflammation of the membrane leads, over many years, to a condition called chronic bronchitis which in due course causes breath-lessness, at first only on exertion but later when resting as well. Inhaling tobacco smoke is one of the chief factors, but our climate and constitution in Britain also contribute to the disease, which is often called the 'English' disease Less frequently, but no less devastatingly, as some later figures will show, the membrane may become cancerous, and the cancer spread throughout the body. This is lung cancer—the major cancer killer of

Western man—whose manifestations are legion, and treatment, except in a small proportion of lucky cases, only palliative. The theories connecting cigarette smoking with lung cancer are discussed later. The constituents of tobacco smoke which contribute most to chest disease are probably the tars. The nicotine and carbon monoxide gas probably contribute most to heart disease.

Nicotine is carried from the lungs by the blood to the adrenal gland and stimulates it to produce a hormone, noradrenaline, which in small quantities increases the amount of fat circulating in the blood vessels and causes them to fur up—the process known as atheroma (or hardening of the arteries). When atheroma occurs in the heart (or coronary arteries) then a heart attack or coronary thrombosis (see Booklet 2) may occur. If the atheroma occurs elsewhere the effects may be equally serious. Increasing the circulation of fats is only one of a number of factors which play a part in the onset of atheroma. Another is the factor which causes the fat to sit on the artery wall, and harden it. Here the carbon monoxide in tobacco smoke plays a part. It is carried in the blood stream by the blood pigment, haemoglobin, whose normal job is to carry oxygen around.

Oxygen is the fuel that all parts of the body require to run on. Carbon monoxide is a poison present in town gas (but not natural gas) and motor exhaust. Death by carbon monoxide poisoning used to be one of the commonest methods of suicide until recently. Its effects in small amounts on the body are twofold. First it occupies a fuel-carrying position but has no value as fuel itself, thereby effectively reducing the fuel supply to the rest of the body. Secondly, we believe that it encourages the laying down of fat in the artery wall and therefore the production of atheroma.

A look at the facts will help the reader to decide why the word believe is used here.

Carbon Monoxide

In the 1960s workers in Copenhagen found that if they fed rats fatty diets and kept half of them in a normal atmosphere and half in an atmosphere containing carbon monoxide, the rats breathing carbon monoxide suffered more severe arterial disease than the other group. Although one must be careful in assuming that what is true for a rat is true for man, it set scientists measuring the carbon monoxide in the blood of smokers and comparing it with non-smokers. At the Medical Centre we examined the blood carbon monoxide level in both patients and staff, and in answer to criticisms that they were a rather select sample of guinea-pigs, we enlisted the co-operation of the local publican and his customers. The results are summarised below.

With each puff on the cigarette a small quantity of carbon monoxide (CO) is absorbed. The quantity of CO in the blood is measured as a percentage of the blood pigment it occupies. People who suffer from town gas poisoning (now quite uncommon since the general use of North Sea gas) pass out when the CO level reaches around forty per cent and die shortly after. The total amount of CO to be absorbed for each cigarette depends upon the make of cigarette, depth of inhalation, and the condition of the smoker's lungs. For an individual the 'boost' in CO level, for each cigarette smoked, can be measured and Figure 3b shows a hypothetical situation of a smoker's CO level throughout the day being gradually boosted with each of the cigarettes he smokes. Notice that in between each smoke the

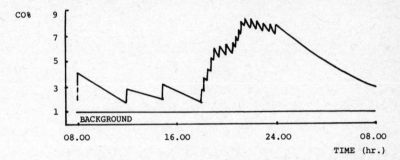

FIG 3b Hypothetical smoker showing his CO level through a typical day.

level is falling. The body removes the poisonous CO through the lungs at a speed which is related to the physical activity of the subject. If he is sedentary then the CO is slowly removed, but if he is running up some stairs or playing squash it is removed much faster. The heavy smoker will boost his CO level with each cigarette until a maximum is reached (which can be as high as twenty per cent but is more usually in the ten to fifteen per cent range) and this again varies from person to person.

Figure 3c shows the kind of differences between people we found among customers in a pub. The left hand column shows the CO level when they entered and the number of cigarettes already smoked. The right hand column shows the CO level when they left the pub and the number of cigarettes smoked in the pub. Some subjects (1–3) had already reached their maximum, but others (4–7) were still pushing the level up. Note subject 8 who was a non-smoker but who was in the smokey atmosphere for three hours. There was no significant change in CO level—most non-smokers living in town have a small amount of CO in the blood, usually between

3.7

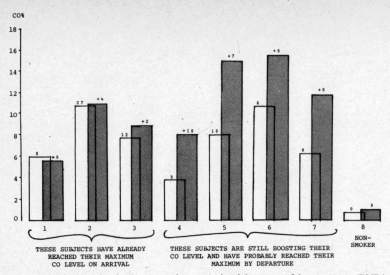

FIG 3c   Individual CO levels taken in a pub on arrival and departure of the customers. (BUPA Medical Centre).

0·1 and 1·0 per cent. One subject achieved a level of sixteen per cent CO by three o'clock in the afternoon—this is one third of the way to unconsciousness!

The next step necessary to interpret these results is to follow up these subjects and see if the high CO levels correlate with the amount of disease diagnosed later in life. If this is so, then with some simple measurements early in life, we will be able to detect the individual in whom smoking is having the most harmful effect and advise him accordingly. For although most of the physiology mentioned so far is either animal work or at its early stage in humans, the statistics that relate smoking to disease which are considered now, will put the experimental work into perspective.

Statistics

It has been known for many years that smokers have a reduced life expectancy. Figure 3d shows the chances of a thirty-five-year-old man reaching retiring age (sixty-five) according to whether or not he smokes. The excess of deaths in smokers seemed to be in lung cancer and heart disease. A study was carried out in the 1950s by Doll and Hill on British doctors—and here the statistical connection between smoking, heart and lung disease became even stronger. Figure 3e shows the excessive occurrence of disease among

3.8

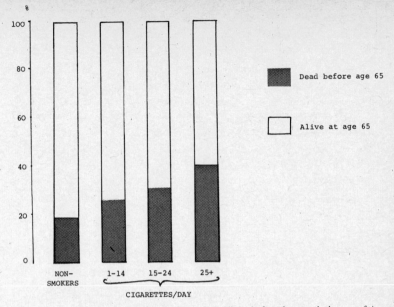

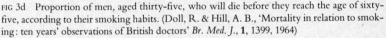

CIGARETTES/DAY

FIG 3d   Proportion of men, aged thirty-five, who will die before they reach the age of sixty-five, according to their smoking habits. (Doll, R. & Hill, A. B., 'Mortality in relation to smoking: ten years' observations of British doctors' *Br. Med. J.*, **1**, 1399, 1964)

the smoking doctors. The study was then continued over the years with even more interesting results. British doctors read the evidence and the majority of smokers gave it up, and this was accompanied by a fall in the amount of chest and heart disease (Figure 3f).

American studies confirm this effect and Figure 3g shows the reduction in heart disease risk when the ex-smoker is compared with the twenty-a-day man. Note that the effect almost totally disappears by the age of sixty-five and over. In the British doctor study it was shown that an ex-smoker of ten years' standing had reduced his chances of lung cancer almost to those of a lifelong non-smoker. The beneficial effect on heart disease from stopping smoking is quicker. It is important to notice, moreover, that non-smokers do occasionally get lung cancer, which reinforces the point, made earlier, that smoking is not the only factor (although probably the most important) concerned with these diseases.

3.9

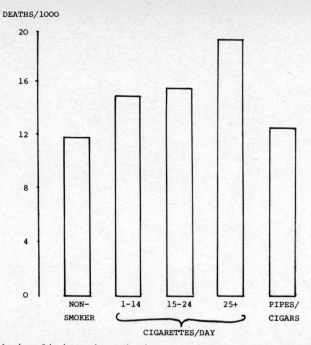

FIG 3e   Number of deaths per thousand each year in male British doctors according to their smoking habits. (Doll, R. & Hill, A. B., 'Mortality in relation to smoking: ten years' observations of British doctors' *Br. Med. J.*, **1**, 1399, 1964)

CAUSE OF DEATH	MALE DOCTORS			ALL MEN (ENGLAND & WALES)		
	PERIOD 1953–57	1962–65	% CHANGE	PERIOD 1953–57	1962–65	% CHANGE
CORONARY HEART DISEASE	294	277	– 6	219	290	+32
LUNG CANCER	60	37	–38	113	120	+ 6
MAJOR DISEASES RELATED TO CIGARETTE SMOKING	539	485	–10	591	633	+ 7
UNRELATED CAUSES	314	262	–17	402	332	–17

FIG 3f   Drop in death rates due to smoking and other causes shown in doctors, compared with the whole population. (Doll, R. & Hill, A. B., 'Mortality in relation to smoking: ten years' observations of British doctors' *Br. Med. J.*, **1**, 1399, 1964)

3.10

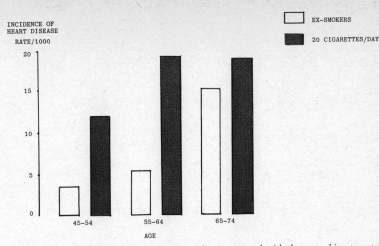

FIG 3g   Reduced risk of heart disease in ex-smokers compared with those smoking twenty a day. Lancet 7/12/74)

Personality and Genetics

Finally in a discussion on the effects of smoking, it is necessary to consider why people smoke. Eminent scientists have attempted to answer this question repeatedly. Smokers tend to have a slightly anxious, neurotic personality. Cigarettes help them to withstand the upsets to their equilibrium that occur daily. One way of demonstrating this physically, was in an American experiment where volunteer smokers were subjected to electric shocks whilst they smoked. The more they smoked, and the higher the nicotine content of the cigarette, the greater the electric shock they could tolerate. Neuroticism represents to some extent an increased susceptibility to the stresses of modern society and for many, smoking counteracts this. Figure 3h shows the percentage of smokers at the Medical Centre according to how many positive answers they give to a question on neuroticism. The more the positive answers, the greater the proportion of smokers. In a similar way, smoking and drinking habits correlate: Figure 3i shows the percentage of smokers at the Medical Centre in each drinking group. Other studies have shown that very heavy drinkers have a high coronary risk, whereas moderate drinkers are a low-risk group. It may be that this effect is due to the different smoking habits of the groups, were it not for the fact that teetotallers are also a high-risk group!

Even more perplexing are the studies carried out on twins to attempt to

NUMBER OF NEUROTIC SYMPTOMS	CIGARETTE SMOKERS (%)	HEAVY DRINKERS (%)
0	28	4.1
1	29	4.6
2	36	6.3
3	36	6.9
4	40	9.0

FIG 3h   Proportion of cigarette smokers and drinkers in patients with neurotic symptoms. (BUPA Medical Centre)

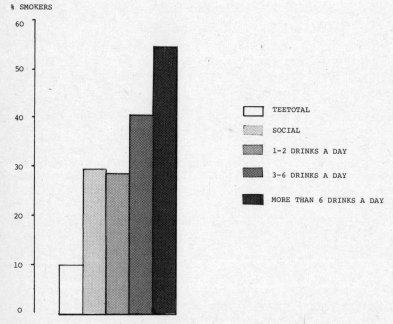

FIG 3i   Proportion of cigarette smokers in each drinking group. (A drink is defined as a single measure of spirits, a glass of wine or half a pint of beer.) (BUPA Medical Centre)

3.12

define a genetic effect on acquiring the smoking habit. Identical twins who had been brought up in different environments were found to resemble each other in their smoking habits more frequently than one would have expected by chance. This work suggested that there was a definite genetic link in the development of smoking habits—maybe even responsible for one-third of factors involved. We know too that there is a hereditary (or genetic) element in many diseases associated with cigarette smoking. This is particularly true for heart disease and it is possible that a genetic proneness to heart disease is accompanied by a similar proneness to take up cigarette smoking. However, this does not explain why there should be a reduction in heart diseases when smoking is stopped.

Thus, the conclusion on cigarette smoking must be that it is clearly associated with a number of diseases, particularly of the lungs and heart, by a variety of mechanisms, all probably playing some part. Furthermore, those who give up smoking find, as time passes, that their likelihood of contracting the disease conforms more to average levels.

Physical Activity

Since the industrial revolution and increasingly still, the Western homo sapiens has become more and more sedentary. With automation and a button-pushing world, physical effort is kept down to a minimum by the majority of people. Physical activity affects fitness and proper functioning of the body. To comprehend the importance of physical activity it is necessary to understand the physiology of exercise.

Physiology

When the body is at rest the heart ticks over at between seventy and ninety beats per minute, pumping blood containing oxygen to all the parts of the body requiring fuel. When the muscles are operating, as they do with any sort of physical activity, they require more oxygen to do their work and the heart speeds up (recognised by an increased pulse rate) and forces out more blood (an increase in work recognised by a rise in blood pressure). These changes are brought about in a number of ways: one of the most important is by the production of adrenalin and like substances, which stimulate the heart to do more work. Initially, at any rate, the action of exercise on the heart resembles closely the effects of smoking a cigarette; here is an interesting paradox, for whereas cigarette smoking is undoubtedly harmful to the heart, exercise is beneficial. This statement is based on a number of facts.

3.13

Most studies about physical activity in man have been based on its relationship to heart disease. It has been noticed for many years by pathologists during autopsy, that marathon and other long distance runners were always remarkably free of atheroma and did not die of heart disease.

In England, surveys comparing bus drivers (sedentary) and bus conductors on double-decker buses (active), showed that the incidence of heart attacks was much less in the conductors. Similarly, a comparison of male telephonists (sedentary) and postmen (active) demonstrated a reduced amount of heart disease in the postmen. Recently, a study showed that the amount of heart trouble in civil servants who took vigorous exercise (this was carefully defined) was less than in those who took none.

Physical activity acts to protect against heart disease in a number of ways. For example, in a smoker it encourages the removal of carbon monoxide from the body rapidly and may minimise the harmful effects. In the civil service study referred to above, the difference in heart disease between smokers and non-smokers was much less in the exercise group, suggesting that a protection mechanism exists in smokers who also take exercise. Regular exercise lowers the resting heart rate. A person with a heart rate in the sixties or below, is fit, which is an advantage for two reasons: first, the heart is more efficient at rest, being able to fulfill body requirements at a lower rate; second, it has more reserve for exercise or emergencies. A man whose resting rate is seventy-two may be able to double that by exercising to 144 (about the maximum for an 'unfit' person), but the man whose rate is sixty will be able to treble the work done by the heart by increasing its rate to 180 (such rates commonly occur in athletes during exercise).

Exercise utilises calories which otherwise might be stored as fat. In other words it helps to keep the weight down. A sedentary existence requires about 2000 calories (or less) in energy, a day, yet the average intake in food is around 3000 calories. Those extra calories in some people are converted to fat and obesity results. A four-minute mile probably uses up 3000 calories of energy and athletes are thin. Physical activity may be a help in reducing weight, but it should not be relied on entirely and many people who take regular exercise when young will find that they have weight problems as they get older and their level of activity falls.

Aches and Pains

A good deal of medical time and energy is devoted to the diagnosis of muscular aches and pains; checking, for instance, that a pain across the chest is not due to heart disease can be an expensive business. If the 1970s man was a fitter specimen, most of these pains would disappear. They arise from underutilised muscles and stiffening joints. A baby can touch the back of his head with his heel or put his toes in his mouth: a ballet dancer or an athlete may maintain such joint mobility, but for the rest of us, lack of use makes ligaments around the joint shorten and produces stiffening. This may cause pain, even when the joint is not used, but it certainly will if the joints are used vigorously but only occasionally. Likewise the muscles lose their power if underused and become flabby. A paunchy man can use his abdominal muscles to keep his paunch in place, but the only time he does so is when he is trying to do his trousers up; from then on he relies on his belt. As time proceeds, underuse of muscles and joints leads to aches and pains causing discomfort, sometimes mimicking serious disease.

Nutrition and Obesity

The old schoolboy adage 'Do you eat to live or live to eat?' contains much sense, particularly so now, when we can divide the world into the over-nourished and the virtually starved. Living our relatively comfortable lives in developed (as distinct from third world) society, we do not realise that obesity can legitimately be described as the commonest disease of developed countries.

Why is over-nutrition a disease?: because we know that thin people live longer than fat people and that in terms of life insurance and other statistics, the overweight carry what is nicely called 'an excess mortality', which means that they do not live so long.

The trouble all starts from the fact that eating is a major pleasure and because of this and because of the availability of high calorie foods, we all eat too much, which is of course why the disease is so common.

Eating Patterns

G. K. Chesterton referred to: 'The portly presence of potentates goodly in girth'. One of the hazards of public life is too many dinners, because 'public display eating' has become one of the rituals of civilised behaviour. Indeed, entertaining friends or celebrating various domestic and other events, all hinge round a major or minor feast.

But in both our public and private lives, we do not realise the extent to which habit and custom determine our eating patterns. Different countries have their own special foods and methods of cooking and within each country socio-economic groups have their own variant of the pattern. Thus, in Britain it is the so-called working class that tend to have chips with everything, even when on the Costa Brava.

This is important because both food intake and the feeling of hunger or the expectation of the next meal, is determined by the social pattern of eating, with regard to quality, quantity and nature of food expected. Thus, dietary behaviour follows a family and a social pattern and constitutes within a group, what is called a shared environmental factor. It is, in fact, seldom that one sees a single fat member of a family; mostly all the family is fat because they all eat too much.

It is now realised that bottle-fed babies are apt to start life too fat: because the artificial milk is not as 'right' as natural breast milk, the mother trying to do her best for the baby, tends firstly to make it up too strong, secondly, to give too much and thirdly, perhaps too often. All this is fostered by the cult of the 'podgy', but bonny baby. However, fat babies make fat children, who become obese adults.

Eating patterns acquired in childhood persist into adult life and then get passed on to the next generation. Thus, not only do 'chips with everything' become an 'inherited' characteristic, but so do the consumption of convenience foods, such as ice cream and sweets.

Physiology of Food

Food provides the energy to keep the body going. Its energy value is measured in calories, and as seen earlier, the sedentary man requires around 2000 calories of fuel a day to fulfill his basic needs. If energy intake is surplus to requirements, it may be stored as fat. When starvation occurs these fat stores are used up, and when exhausted the body runs out of fuel and dies.

Food constituents are divided into three groups:

Carbohydrate   Comes as sugar, flour and starchy products as in bread, potatoes and rice. One gram produces four calories, and they are relatively cheap and palatable and tend to get consumed in great quantity.
Protein   Found mainly in the flesh of animals, i.e. meat and fish. Also present in eggs, milk, cheese and other dairy products. Provides four calories per gram in energy terms and is the most expensive of foods.
Fats   Greasy food characterised by butter or fat bacon. Meat is either lean or fatty according to how much fat it contains. Dairy products are also rich in fat. It provides nine calories per gram.

Most foods consist of a mixture of these elements, and when eaten, these complex chemicals that make up food are dissolved by the digestive juices of the stomach and small intestines, and broken down into their component parts which are chemically much smaller and can be transferred from the intestine to the liver and other parts of the body in the blood stream. They are then reassembled into the chemicals that the body requires. The whole process is called metabolism and during it body fat is produced, not only from the components of the dietary fat, but also from the components of dietary carbohydrate. In other words sugar and starch, which are basic carbohydrates, if not used for body building or fuelling, may be changed into fat. The components into which dietary fat is split are called 'fatty acids', and during metabolism these are reconstructed into a variety of substances, one of the most important being cholesterol. Cholesterol is a starting point for many important hormones which keep the body running smoothly, but too much of it can be harmful, and it is a major contributory factor to heart disease (see Booklet 2).

Minerals and Vitamins

As well as the main food types described above, the body requires water, minerals and vitamins. In any civilised society, diet is balanced to include a satisfactory amount of all of them. If, for instance, vitamins are destroyed in the process of making a foodstuff, the manufacturer may be obliged to make good the loss before marketing the product. This applies particularly to white bread, which is as nutritious as brown bread because the vital elements destroyed in the baking are restored at a later stage. The important minerals and vitamins are as follows:

Iron The body contains enough iron to make a four-inch nail. It is essential for the blood pigment, and shortage of it causes anaemia.
Calcium The bony skeleton of the body is made up of complex calcium chemicals, deficiency causes softening and weakening of the bones, leading to fractures.
Vitamins These are divided into two groups according to whether or not they dissolve in water. Vitamins B and C are water soluble, and consist of a number of chemicals, deficiency of which leads to diseases such as beri-beri, pellagra and scurvy. They are contained in fresh vegetables and fruit. Other vitamins are found in fatty products, which is why we force cod-liver oil down children's throats. Vitamin D is the most important, for this controls the growth of bones, and without it they do not develop correctly, giving rise to rickets.

Deficiency of minerals and vitamins in our society develops mainly because the body is over-utilising them, as in children with growing bones, or pregnant or nursing women, who are feeding for two, or in elderly people who neglect their diet and possibly don't absorb the minerals as well as they ought to. In these groups of people special attention must be paid to their diet, but in other healthy people there is no proven benefit in swallowing vitamin pills, and disease due to excess indulgence in this habit has been described.

There are two other important factors in diet and nutrition: one is bulk and the other palatability. The digestive system, which is designed to extract the good and the valuable from food, and expell the residue, does also need 'bulk', to grind on, as it were. Thus, one can get the essentials plus calories in a very concentrated form, as might be used in space flights, but this would lead to constipation. Much of what we eat in vegetables and cereal particularly, is indigestible bulk or fibre. But this is essential to keep the flow of solids through the digestive tract and to stop constipation. Some experts say that third world diets, because they contain so much fibre, protect against spastic colon and cancers.

Palatability is much more subjective and depends to a degree on fashion, but there is no doubt that since 1900, rising standards of living have led to an increased consumption of animal fats (Figure 3j), and sugar—where consumption per person per day has risen from around 90 grams to 130 grams. The advent of pre-fabricated convenience foods has made it easy to eat a high calorie diet. This is helped by the fact that carbohydrates and fats are (relatively) cheap.

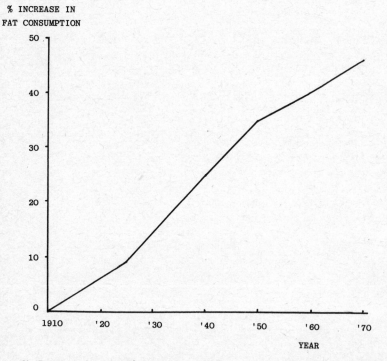

FIG 3j Percentage increase in fat consumption this century (National Food Survey, 1974)

3.18

Body Build, Personality and Weight

Experts divide us into three main 'somato-types' of body build: the tall, thin, rather manic and active ectomorph, who is the lucky chap who can eat anything and everything and never put on weight; the muscular, thick-set mesomorph who is heavy, but not necessarily fat, but who may run to fat when he gives up using his muscles; and the pear-drop man, the endo-morph who is rounded and mostly with fat.

Obviously, we do not all fall precisely into these categories, but the body build does give a good guide as to what weight ought to be. Obviously, too, people of roughly the same height are built differently, so that the more thick-set person will have a higher normal weight than a thin person. And most weight tables reflect this.

Another difference between people is the rate at which they burn up energy. Manic active ectomorphs seem to use up energy more effectively than the good converters, who stack it away as fat. It is the good converters who have to watch their weight.

We have already made the point about character, discipline and weight control and there is a group of people who genuinely find this difficult. Eating is such a basic activity that it would be surprising if it was not related to equally basic psychological reactions. Some people when they feel insecure and anxious, tend to over-eat, they are eating for comfort and security. A lot of seriously fat people do have a personality disturbance, which drives them to stuff themselves. Many of them are unhappy, in-secure and isolated people. And in medical terms, it is very difficult to help them. They can be brought into hospital and literally starved, but the moment they go back into the world, they start over-eating again. In fact, they are rather tragic characters.

Assessing Weight

As has been implied, it is surplus fat rather than bone and muscle, that concerns us. Fat is mostly stored under the skin so that skin thickness is a good rough measure of obesity. But in practice, fat people do just look fat and it is not really very difficult to judge them.

Body build apart, weight can be judged in two ways: first, the average for the group or population; and second, the desirable, which is based on survival figures from life insurance experience. Average weights can be misleading, because obviously, if the whole group is overweight, the average will be high and they will all carry excess mortality. Again, and this is what has happened since the war, as standards of nutrition and over-nutrition go up, so does the average weight.

Thus, an average weight compares you with your fellows, and there is a socio-economic difference here. For instance, there is now some evidence that social classes IV and V, the semi-skilled and manual workers are less disciplined about diet than those in classes I and II. Women tend to be more weight-conscious than men and are more prone to diet etc.

Desirable weights, however, give you the right target to aim at for survival; they are a bit of a statistical guess, but do get one more or less into the target area. They should, in our view, be interpreted in relation to other findings. Thus, a person with a long-lived family, low blood pressure and who does not smoke cigarettes, can probably afford to be a bit heavier than a moderately hypertensive cigarette smoker. Sensible medical judgement comes into advising on the weight target.

Living Sensibly— Practical Advice

Most intelligent people reading and understanding the facts presented here, must by now be convinced of the danger of cigarette smoking, obesity and inactivity. Altering habits of a lifetime is not easy and there is no point in prolonging a life made miserable by not doing most of the things that one enjoys. Looking at the evidence in perspective, there is no doubt that cigarette smoking is by far the most dangerous habit of the seventies and practical advice must start with this.

Smoking

Don't think in terms of giving up cigarettes *but of taking up non-smoking*. Being a non-smoker becomes a way of life; just as smoking when you started at school was the 'clever' thing to do, so now as an adult, taking up non-smoking is the clever and hard thing to do. There are several methods of giving up—and the personality of the individual must choose—but first they must be motivated. Re-read the statistics. Go to the pub in the morning and listen to the smokers coughing. Talk to lift operators in big buildings—the people that look seventy but are only fifty-five, who cannot walk more than a few paces because they become breathless. When you visit friends in hospital, glance at the others—half of them are there because of smoking—and on your way out pass the mortuary and think of the ones who dropped dead suddenly in their prime. If this does not motivate you, then you are demonstrating the typical addict's trait of deceiving yourself. But, once there is sufficient motivation, 'stop', just like that. If you are a gambling man take a bet with a colleague who is also giving up: say the first to start again pays the other £100. Once you stop, you become a non-smoker, part of an elite group, proud to belong to it, to be able to smell again, and having got rid of that cough in the morning. Initially, it will not be easy. If you have been a heavy smoker you may suffer from withdrawal symptoms, and intense craving, depression, restlessness and insomnia and other physical symptoms. These will pass in a few days and are often psychological, rather than true withdrawal symptoms. Distract yourself—by taking exercise, talking, walking, being a little manic for a few days, doing the things around the house you have been meaning to do for years. Keep away from places where smoking is encouraged for the first few days, seek the company of non-smokers and adopt the holier-than-thou attitude with smokers. Tell them they smell, which they do, but it may take six months or more before your own sense of smell improves sufficiently to detect it. Your friends and family will implore you to take it up again—call you bad-tempered and worse. Explain that it is only temporary, beg their indulgence, spend the money you are saving on presents for them, for the irritability will pass in a matter of days. What may never pass, and which is often the downfall of the well-motivated 'non(ex-)smoker', is the craving. Even after ten or more years of non-smoking one hears remarks like 'I'm dying for a cigarette'. The actual crave only lasts a short time—talk about it—do something different—anything that breaks your train of thought— and the 'crave' will pass.

If this is impossible, keep a stock of the largest, most expensive havana cigars, light one up and satisfy your crave. The important thing is that you should not inhale, hence the need for getting the strongest. It is no use turning to a small cheroot, which is just the same as smoking the strongest cigarette. Sometimes a smelly pipe is a good alternative for the craving, in the early days. This really foul habit requires pockets full of equipment to maintain the small inferno, produces an acrid smoke that even pipe-smokers rarely inhale, and takes so long to get going, that the crave may have worn off by that time! However, all the evidence shows that cigars and pipe-smoking are much less damaging to health, if not inhaled.

So now you are a non-smoker; set a proud example to your children; travel in and campaign for non-smoking compartments on trains, in theatres and restaurants, and for smoking advertisements to be abolished. Make non-smoking a positive thing—a way of life.

Exercise

This is the point to start thinking about the amount of exercise you take. The big enemies of fitness are the motor car and the job. Apart from the stressful aspects of motoring, it is so convenient that it often reduces the amount of basic exercise to a minimum. It need not be so: walk to the station twice a week (and back again, don't forget). In summer do it more often. Park the car several blocks away if you are a city driver. Buy a bicycle, either a cheap one to be used occasionally when the weather is good, or a fold up one, which can easily be put in the back of a taxi if a storm breaks.

Most managerial jobs are sedentary. Do not allow yourself to be convinced that walking around a factory plant or to other people's offices is good exercise—it only is if you become breathless (assuming you have no lung or heart disease already). Walk up all stairs: this helps and also gives you an indication of how fit you are; if you are panting by the second flight, you need a medical check-up and more exercise. Get a dog, a large one that needs exercising, not a small one that stops at every lamp-post. Garden at weekends and in the evenings and make sure you get a little breathless doing it. In town go to a well-run gymnasium instead of the pub at lunchtime. Such exercise should be graded, and in a good gymnasium it is, so that you do not strain your puny muscles at first.

It is never too late to improve fitness, although a medical check-up may be sensible. Similarly, there is no ideal form of exercise—do what you enjoy or least dislike. Books are available for exercise schedules, usually done at home, but they are not the most effective. Golf can be exercise but it does have other hazards, particularly the club bar. Older people should be careful to compete with others of their own age and an activity schedule should contain three main points:

1. Putting bones and joints through their full range of movements every day.
2. Developing and maintaining muscle strength by press-ups and other exercises. Backs are very prone to be painful, if not regularly exercised.
3. Make the heart work and develop a reserve. This involves getting breathless every day.

Weight

Weight control consists of calorie book-keeping: one needs to get into a break-even situation where the weight remains steady, but at roughly the right level.

Thus, someone who is overweight has two problems: the first is to lose weight until they get down to bogey; and the second is to rebalance at the right level. This means developing a new eating habit which will become part of your life and after a couple of months you will no longer miss the sugar in your tea and the mid-morning biscuit. What this also means—and this is critical to the whole situation—is that crash starvation courses are little long-term help.

We always advise that budgetting should be over a week and not just a

3.22

day. Thus, a busy businessman who has a bad week of lunches and dinners must 'bant' over the weekend in order to break even. But within this, and the great point about eating out is that there is choice, and by sticking to non-fatty foods, like steak and salad, one can do reasonably well.

There has been a vogue recently for appetite suppressant pills. These do sometimes help, particularly in the early stages, but they are not without danger, particularly if taken long-term. Medical advice should be sought, and in any case, the effective ones require a prescription.

Basically, and as with smoking, there is no real substitute for resolve. The rules are as follows:

1. Get the co-operation of your wife: if you lunch out or eat in a canteen, work towards a light supper. She does not necessarily need to go on demonstrating what a good cook she is.
2. Treat calories like pennies—and the pounds will look after themselves. This means no sugar in the tea and coffee, no nibbling between meals, 'dry' drinks rather than sweet ones, no second helpings, small portions rather than large ones, low calorie fillers, tonic and bitter lemon for drinks etc.
3. Learn to pick and choose: eating is a major pleasure and you are entitled to eat the things you like and leave out those you don't. If you want your calories in alcohol—fine, but don't have bread and potatoes as well. Carbohydrate foods—bread, potatoes, jam, cakes, puddings etc.—are pleasant to eat, but high calorie. They are the easiest to cut out. If you adore puddings, allow yourself three a week and leave out spuds.
4. Budget for a blow out: again, eating is a social and personal pleasure so allow yourself occasional indulgencies—it's all good fun and provided you break even in the week, all will remain well.
5. Take plenty of exercise, it gives you a good margin, but remember that beer after rugby probably lands you up on calorie credit—hence the size of most rugby players.
6. Weigh yourself once a week at the same time of day and don't let your weight creep up.

Diets

These really are ten-a-penny and there is little but faith and recommendation in choosing between them. They all work by helping you to eat less. How this is achieved is immaterial, except that it is wise to finish up with an eating pattern that is compatible with your way of life. The one we recommend, given at the end of this booklet, is based on common sense and easy understanding and it has worked for our patients for over twenty years.

3.23

The important thing is to understand what you are trying to achieve and then bend the rules to keep happy. On this diet a significantly overweight person should lose a pound a day for the first couple of weeks, which is most encouraging. Obviously, the final loss is harder and slower, but by then you should be used to the diet and it will not appear so hard.

Basically, this is a high protein, moderate fat, low carbohydrate diet. Hunger in this situation is best dealt with by low calorie, bulky foods, like vegetables, salad, fruit etc. In fact, apples and carrots for nibbling can be a great help. Eggs in moderation (up to three a week) are fine, unless the blood cholesterol is raised. But the daily fried egg and bacon, the Englishman's staple diet, is one of the highest cholesterol meals there is!

Weight Watchers is an organisation which works a bit like Alcoholics Anonymous, but they are far from anonymous. The organisation offers two things: first, a perfectly sensible and 'livable-on' diet; and second, group solidarity to get you going and keep you on the straight and narrow. It is mostly for women, but we did have a man who lost three stones with them and became their star pupil. They have groups in most areas and have recently produced a good cookery book. If you want a weekly weigh-in, this is very much for you.

Finally, do not only apply sensible nutrition to yourself—start indoctrinating your children. The commonest infectious disease in the civilised world is dental caries, caused by bad nutrition in childhood, leading to false teeth and unhealthy mouths in young adulthood. A child will benefit greatly from a sensible attitude to food, particularly sweets and lollipops!

Special Diets

These are usually much more rigorous and are indicated because of specific diseases. The commonest is for diabetes, followed probably by low cholesterol diets.

Diabetes is a disease, mostly found in its mild forms in middle- and older age. It is commoner in overweight people and arises from an inability to deal with carbohydrate metabolism. Mild diabetes, which produces sugar in the urine, can usually be dealt with by diet alone; more severe forms may require 'pills' as well as diet; and the most serious form needs regular insulin injections to replace the hormone which is not working or not available. Basically a diabetic diet excludes most carbohydrate but allows fat and protein.

Low cholesterol diets are prescribed for those in danger of arteriosclerosis because of high blood fats. They tend to be boring because they exclude animal fats and dairy products, but as coronary thrombosis is a killing disease, the diet, which may be aided by certain drugs, is worth tolerating.

Other conditions which may need long-term dieting are: kidney disease—low salt diet; gout—mainly the avoidance of foods containing uric acid; and several serious metabolic disturbances found in children. Allergies, too, mean avoiding the substances to which the individual is sensitive—be these eggs or shell-fish. All these conditions need to be dealt with under strict medical supervision.

Conclusion

The advice outlined here is the ideal. It should be emphasised that it is not worth making your life longer if it is going to be miserable. If you really cannot become a non-smoker, cut down, change to a milder brand in terms of tar and nicotine content and smoke less of each cigarette, leaving a large stub where some of the noxious chemicals are trapped. As for exercise, take every opportunity to walk rather than ride and you will be half way to fitness. Any sensible man can control his calorie input over a week and still enjoy food. Just losing half a stone makes clothes fit better and the subject feel fitter. Physically and mentally improved you should live to enjoy a healthy retirement.

Appendix A

AverageWeights at Different Ages and Heights

Height	Under 30 M	Under 30 F	30–39 M	30–39 F	40–49 M	40–49 F	50–59 M	50–59 F	60+ M	60+ F	Height
4'11"	—	115	—	121	—	128	—	131	—	133	4'11"
5 ft.	—	117	—	123	—	130	—	133	—	135	5 ft.
5'1"	—	119	—	125	—	132	—	136	—	138	5'1"
5'2"	—	121	—	127	—	135	—	139	—	142	5'2"
5'3"	134	124	138	130	141	138	142	142	139	145	5'3"
5'4"	136	127	142	134	145	141	146	145	143	148	5'4"
5'5"	141	131	146	138	149	145	150	149	146	152	5'5"
5'6"	144	134	150	142	154	149	155	152	152	154	5'6"
5'7"	148	138	154	146	158	153	159	157	156	159	5'7"
5'8"	151	142	158	150	162	157	163	162	161	164	5'8"
5'9"	156	146	163	154	167	161	168	166	166	168	5'9"
5'10"	160	150	167	158	171	164	173	171	171	175	5'10"
5'11"	165	154	172	160	176	168	178	175	176	179	5'11"
6 ft.	170	158	176	164	180	171	182	179	181	186	6 ft.
6'1"	175	—	181	—	185	—	187	—	186	—	6'1"
6'2"	179	—	186	—	190	—	192	—	191	—	6'2"
6'3"	183	—	192	—	196	—	198	—	197	—	6'3"

Note: Desirable weights are roughly equivalent to mean weights under 30

Appendix B

Correction of Overweight

Obesity is caused by storage of surplus calories; weight loss always ensues if calorie intake becomes less than calorie expenditure. You can hasten loss of weight both by cutting down consumption of dispensable sources of energy (carbohydrate, fat and alcohol) and by increased physical activity. Depending how fit you are, you should walk for an additional half-hour a day (equivalent to loss of a stone a year), or jog, or swim, or play competitive sport; the important point is to do so daily or as often as possible. If dieting for more than six weeks, take a vitamin tablet twice daily, and have a regular medical check.

You will quickly adapt to a calorie-restricted diet. Hunger is seldom a problem after the first two to three days; if you find you need to eat late in the evening, choose from the following *minimum-calorie foods*:

Clear soup (skim if necessary)
Salads (no potato, no avocado); dress with lemon juice
Grilled mushrooms
Grapefruit (try grilling it)
Green vegetables
Tea or coffee with or without skimmed milk and saccharin
Tonic water, tomato-juice, dietetic squash
Marmite, Bovril

You may eat the following amounts of *protein and calorie-containing foods* (one day's allowance):

4 oz. lean poultry or meat: *or* 10 oz. grilled or steamed fish; *or* 8oz. cottage cheese
1/3 oz. butter, margarine
3 very thin slices of bread or 5 crisp-breads or dry biscuits
2 rashers of very lean grilled bacon
2 apples or oranges or peaches or pears, or 1 banana, or 15 grapes or cherries or 10 strawberries (unsweetened)

And supplement your meals freely from the minimum-calorie list. You may also have three eggs a week and half a pound (raw weight) of potatoes a week—boiled or baked in jackets.

You should *avoid items on this list*—if you don't, the dieting will take much longer:

Sugars, jams, honey, chocolates and sweets
Visible fat on meat or bacon
Cakes, sweet biscuits, cereals and porridge
Cream, mayonnaise, thickened gravy
Thick soups
Nuts, dried fruit
Ice cream
Alcohol, cocoa, sweetened soft drinks unless calorie-free

Cooking

Grilling and steaming are preferable. Avoid fried and roast foods.

Weight

Record your weight, in minimal clothing, on rising. You may lose eight to ten pounds a month. If you consistently lose less than one pound a week, you are still eating to excess.

Dining Out

Stay as close as possible to the instructions in the three lists. Compensate by eating less the day before. Choose grapefruit or a seafood (avoid all dressings). Pick grilled lean meat or fish, end with fruit and coffee. Don't waste a week's hard dieting with a blow-out.

3.28

Appendix C

Modified–Fat, Low Cholesterol Diet

This diet is designed to reduce the amount of fatty substances, including cholesterol, in your blood. Intake of hard ('saturated') fats—mainly animal fats—is restricted and these are partly replaced by soft ('polyunsaturated') fats and oils; intake of cholesterol itself is also reduced. You will find that you can eat well while adhering to these principles.

Meat and fish

Restrict fatty meats to six to eight ounces a week (mutton, lamb, pork and pork products, goose and duck). Choose fish, or lean poultry or meat (chicken, turkey, veal, hare) wherever possible, allowing six to eight ounces a day. Fish may be dry or fatty; tuna, salmon, mackerel are acceptable. Grilling, or frying in recommended oil, are preferable; when roasting, place meat on a rack to allow its fat to drain. Restrict liver, kidneys, sweetbread, tongue, sausages and shellfish; avoid brains and fish roe. Trim all visible fat off meat. Order mince prepared from trimmed lean meat.

Dairy Produce, Margarine, Eggs

Avoid butter as spread and in cooking. Avoid whole milk and cream. Restrict most cheeses to one to one-and-a-half ounces a week; Edam is relatively low in fat, and skimmed-milk cheeses are satisfactory. Use skimmed milk freely (dried or liquid). Use margarines rich in polyunsaturated fat (such as Flora) freely as spread and in baking and frying. Limit egg yolks to two weekly (white may be used freely). Avoid non-dairy coffee-creamers. And avoid all ice-creams except sorbet.

Fruit, Vegetables, Nuts

Almost all are acceptable, and walnuts and almonds are rich in unsaturated fat. Avoid coconut and restrict peanuts.

Cooking

Use sunflower oil, corn oil or safflower oil for frying and roasting, and in salad dressing and marinades. Avoid hard cooking fats.

Prepared Foods

Most commercial biscuits, cakes and desserts contain saturated fat; so do chocolates, fudge and toffee. Most bread and cereals are low in fat. Avoid potato crisps. Sugar contains no fat. Bake at home with allowed margarines or oils.

Dining Out

Chinese and fish restaurants are ideal. Elsewhere, regard all fat-containing items as likely to be rich in saturated fat. Select clear soup, or asparagus. Follow with fish, selected poultry or lean meat, or a pasta (grilled meat is preferable). End with a sorbet or fruit. Balance an enforced dietary lapse by extra care the next day or two. And enjoy your wine—it's harmless in moderation.

Acknowledgements

To the Royal College of Physicians for permission to use Figures 3d, 3e and 3f. To the landlord and customers of the Tollington Arms, Hornsey Road, London for submitting two samples of blood each, upon which the data presented in Figure 3c are based.

4
A Woman's Life

H. Beric Wright, MB, FRCS

Introduction

Some years ago we went to a Greek Island on what was my wife's first 'far Mediterranean' tour. Driving through the country and then the villages in the local bus, my wife became increasingly angry by the realisation that the women seemed to be doing all the work, while the men sat about in the cafés playing cards and backgammon. This reminded me of the years I spent in South-East Asia after the war and my first visit to Hong Kong, where I saw 'little women' dressed in black, almost drowned in their shady straw hats, swarming up and down the bamboo scaffolding of a new office block—carrying seemingly heavy loads of building material. Indeed, in some parts of the world, women appear to be able to work physically just as hard as men and for just as long.

In Europe, for instance, it is usual to make a fuss about pregnancy and a woman will traditionally have considerable time off, both before and after the event. Peasant societies cannot afford this luxury; often the baby is born at work, bundled up and taken into the field. Hygiene and living standards apart, there is no evidence that either mother or child is any the worse for this seemingly brutal treatment. On the contrary, because she is physically fit and has neither the time nor the tradition to worry about 'female ailments', the chances are that she is much healthier than her Western counterpart.

Again many years ago, I talked with a very distinguished woman industrial medical officer, who had been asked at the beginning of the war to advise the US Government on physical work limitations for women. The more she thought about this and discovered what peasant women could do, the less she was convinced that the 'all American woman' needed 'Factories Act Protection'.

Traditionally women are regarded as the weaker sex, but as I have implied, the evidence for this is mythological rather than factual. In our society, women have an appreciably lower death rate and slightly longer life expectancy—at all ages. Statistically this means that there are more women than men in the population, particularly in the middle and older age-groups. Men die off sooner, largely from coronary thrombosis, leaving widows either to flourish or languish on their own; or perhaps to think about further marriage. Thus, we can take it that women are inherently tough, verge on the indestructable, capable of hard and sustained physical work, present in greater numbers than men—but yet in Western society, down-trodden, mildly depressed, queueing up in doctors' surgeries with backache and general misery and agitating for liberation by legislation.

Being a mere, if sympathetic male, brought up in an environment of equality and working women (my mother is a distinguished gynaecologist

4.3

who is credited by her friends as being the one person they know who has brought up four 'only' children) not only have I been concerned to encourage women to pull their weight, but unable to understand why they don't or haven't. Statistically one would expect there to be just as many women painters, musicians, composers, politicians and so on, as there are men. But no, writing apart, women have not made the artistic grade and are now reduced to moaning extensively about their inferior role and asking Parliament and UNO to protect them with legislation. This is in fact, being written during International Women's Year and at the time of Mrs Thatcher's Tory succession. I hope that between the two, women will negotiate a better deal with society at large.

I suspect that what has happened is that historically Western man has 'conned' his mate into accepting her biological purpose as an unpaid mum and nursemaid, etc. Obviously a lot of women like this, but there are no inherent reasons, except behavioural tradition, why dad should not look after the young, while mum goes out to work. In some spheres of activity, the economic arguments in favour of doing this may be overwhelming. Competent and indeed even less competent secretaries, can get appreciable salaries, which are often well above those offered to male clerical workers doing just as responsible work.

Victorian middle-class mothers brought their daughters up to be a bit fragile and to expect sex to be joyless, menstruation painful and childbirth a burden. As they tended to have flocks of ill-paid servants, the ladies suffered excrutiatingly from boredom and a wide range of psychosomatic diseases. The equivalent working-class man appears to have turned his wife into a drudge who was lucky to be taken out once a week, while he spent most of his evenings at the boozer or in the working man's club.

Mercifully and at far too long last, all this is now rapidly changing and the roles and priorities within marriage are altering towards more equality of relationship. Women now have a much wider range of emotional and physical choice, much of which stems from removal of the fear of pregnancy following sexual contact. The nature of marriage is altering—I am sure on the whole for the better—partly because of the need for a joint income when setting up a home and partly because it is now the norm for the better-educated school-leaving girl, to do something which is both gainful and useful—if not always satisfying and amusing. Because of all this, I would expect women to become healthier and happier, but as happiness stems from a number of factors, which are not always fully realised or thought through, it is perhaps worth looking at some of the problem areas from the point of view of the woman.

Adult life starts with the genetic and environmental inheritance donated by parents. Here it is worth noting that many later problems stem from what is now loosely called the generation gap—a catch phrase arising from parental inability to communicate with, or influence their adolescent children. Children require a stable and sensible background, knowledge about behaviour and sexual matters—including contraception and some standards of behaviour. It is desirable that this knowledge should be acquired formally from school or parent and not from the grapevine of the school gossip group and the inuendo of salacious publications. Thus, better or worse equipped, the youngster moves to work or further training and perhaps too soon, may get married and then may or may not continue working.

Marriage, middle age (whether this be married or single), and finally retirement, each produce problem areas which may be worth separate consideration. Most of the problems arise from relationships or the lack of them, so that much of this booklet will be about relationships and the effect that these have on health. There are also some specifically 'female' medical problems, which will also be discussed.

Growing Up and Leaving Home

As has already been said, the modern tendency is for the sixteen- to seventeen-year-old girl to make a fairly smooth transition from school to work, via either 'in-house' training, in industry or commerce, or an overt training course at a secretarial college or similar institution. Others may go to the university, to teacher training, to nursing, or other caring professions. The main problem seems to be deciding what to do and being sufficiently motivated to overcome the initial disappointments and disciplines of establishing a new and adult identity. The more professional the training, the better the final identity. But vocations, like nursing and teaching, require a great deal of emotional maturity to survive the course and in the case of the former the very hard work, discipline and irregular hours involved.

Depending a bit on age, maturity and domestic background, leaving school and going to work or training, provides an opportunity to get away from home and be an adult on one's own. With a little help and encouragement, it is now not too difficult for a youngster to get established in a flat with two or three others and to have a cheerful social life. Even if it is not essential to leave home, I suspect that one can generalise and say that it is highly desirable that a youngster should. It is far more difficult, for parents and children, to establish an adult relationship if they remain too involved with each other domestically. Parents always tend to disapprove of their children's growing-up behaviour and the less they know about it, the less alarmed they will be. Week-ends can well be enough for both parties and on this basis they might even enjoy the contact.

It seems very difficult for parents, particularly mothers, to get away from wanting their children to remain dependent and grateful. Psychologically, they appear to be trying to buy dependence and gratitude by continuing to provide, they then become 'hurt' when their activity elicits the wrong response. Also, many rather lonely mums appear to have little else to do but worry disapprovingly about children and grandchildren. And this is a poor basis for an adult relationship. Similarly, I believe that the young should be brought up to pull their domestic weight and not be looked after and provided for too much. I am sure that this makes them better wives and husbands.

My mother, with her lifetime of experience of women and their problems, used to say that it was the most over-protected girls who fell hardest and whose mums were most outraged by the 'bump'. The young debutante (who mercifully hardly exists now) whose first contact with predatory males might be in the ski-hut or taxi-seat, was 'easy game' and often became pregnant. Biologically animals expell their young from the nest or burrow. I suspect that humans should do the same: over-protection can be disastrous.

Every young person, hopefully from fifteen or sixteen onwards, has to start making up their mind about their attitude to sexual stimulation. Hopefully, their parents and the community of which they are part, will give them standards and knowledge, so that they know what they are doing and do not get unreasonably caught. A major part of growing up consists of learning to live with sexuality, objectively and without guilt. Similarly parents and daughters have now to decide if and when to go on the Pill, and it is perhaps wise to be safe rather than sorry.

Pre-war morality was based on biblical traditions of virgin marriage, at least for women. Young men were allowed to cut their teeth on rather dubious young or not so young ladies, but 'nice' girls were expected to remain intact. Intact they may have been, but ignorant they also were—which could be equally disastrous.

All learning is by acquiring experience and sexuality has to be experienced to be controlled and understood. There is no evidence that pre-marital intercourse destroys or harms subsequent marriage to a different partner, and one can advance the supposition that the more experience that goes into a marital decision, the better the decision is likely to be. To quote my mother again (and for the last time): when she started her Family Planning work in the late 1920s, she was appalled by the small proportion of patients who enjoyed their sex. Thirty years later, the opposite was nearly true, in that many women were setting out—sub-

4.6

consciously—to castrate their men by being over-demanding. But against this, one must not lose sight of the fact that the more traditional view of marriage works (or appears to) reasonably well. It would be interesting to know over the past fifty years, the proportion of people who marry without previous sexual experience. A social class breakdown would add further fascination to the figures. The main point is that marriage may be improved rather than harmed by premarital intercourse.

I believe that the early years of work after school are vital to the growing up process. During this time, the adolescent has to learn to stand on his or her own feet, to gain emotional and sexual experience and to become an independent person who knows where they are going. Only then in my view, should marriage be contemplated and, hopefully, delayed as long as possible. This complicated and often necessarily traumatic process is best done away from home and in a peer group who can learn from and discuss with each other. Obviously a stable home base with wise, sympathetic and understanding parents is an enormous help. But parents must aim at establishing an adult independent relationship and deny themselves the luxury of trying to turn their young into images of themselves. This is, of course, much easier to preach than to achieve.

Secretary Birds and Others— The Young Working Girl

I have two sons, both of whom are now doctors, and in my early days at the Institute of Directors Medical Centre, I used to try to encourage them to take an interest in the super girls who worked for us. Apart from being naturally suspicious of 'father's choice', they used also to say 'Look Dad. They are out of our class: students can only afford students and nurses. We can't live with the (then) £20-a-week girl.'

A youngster leaving secretarial school, etc. can now have a gorgeous time. She is pretty well paid, can shop around until she finds a congenial job and can enjoy a reasonably full social life. By getting into a group, she learns how to deal with the 'work group' and to pull her weight in the office. She has to accept a certain amount of discipline and to be supervised. She should also learn how to look after herself, socially, which includes cooking, cleaning, budgeting and emotional and physical self-preservation. As has already been said, she must set her own standards of sexual behaviour and learn how much she wants and can manage in the way of alcoholic intake. Again one can only learn about alcohol by experience, but young girls who have drunk too much are extremely vulnerable as their defences are down—men do use drink as a trap—and they are more easily flattered by older men (e.g. at the office party). It must also be remembered that alcohol, like nicotine, is a drug of addiction and women who drink too much probably get a worse social reputation than men, i.e. there may be a double standard of behaviour here.

As the secretary progresses up the ladder, she has to learn about keeping confidences, managing and being managed and relationships with her immediate boss. These are by definition both complicated and personal. The nature of the job demands close contact and mutual esteem. The temptations are enormous and pitfalls for both are prodigious. Some of the problems may be created by the fact that many marriages go through difficult or 'flat periods' and the excitement of a new experience may be too tempting. Because of the close contact involved in the work relationship, there is likely to be much more emotional involvement than with a casual liaison on a business trip. A lot of second marriages, too, arise from this situation, but on the whole only when the first marriage was doomed anyway. What is essential in dealing with a complicated situation is a degree of clear-headedness on both sides, so that the consequences of any relationship may be thought out in advance. It may also be sensible for the wife to have good and friendly contact with the office.

Early Marriage

I suspect that there is a tendency, in relation to our current life-style, for people to get married too young. I get worried when I read in the papers about eighteen-year-olds marrying sixteen- or seventeen-year-olds and wonder how these marriages can last. Marriage may be the socially accepted behaviour pattern for most people and obviously it mostly works. In addition, because divorce is so much easier—and, in my view, rightly so—it is now relatively easy to 'give up' an unsatisfactory marriage. But as has already been implied, successful and sound relationships need a great deal of maturity and insight if they are to endure for thirty or forty years. The more individuals have developed or know or have revealed, what sort of people they are going to be, the higher the chances of making the right choice. A couple marrying much before they are, say 25, are just as likely to develop in different directions, as they are to grow together.

There is another factor, which is particularly true of business and some professional people, and this is that if the man is able and ambitious, his career development often leaves little time and energy for emotional and domestic priorities. Unless she is very careful, the wife of such a man may well be left long hours at home with little to do. Professor Pahl of Canterbury and his wife, who have done some sociological studies in this area, suggest that the best wife for a businessman is likely to be someone who has worked in industry or commerce at about his level, i.e. a good secretary will know what his problems are and be able to both talk about and help with them.

Hopefully, the first year or two of marriage—and this is a personal view—will be without children and will be devoted to setting up house, getting to know each other and developing careers. During this time, most things should be shared, including the domestic chores and income. I am a great believer in joint bank accounts with the woman retaining control of at least some of her own money. For instance, it could be a sensible idea to have both joint and private accounts, so that both people have a degree of independence. I know a youngish couple with rather a mean husband who expects his wife to buy the drink for a dinner party out of her earnings. Indeed, she provides most of the housekeeping money. This seems a bit hard—but real meanness is a fascinating quirk of behaviour about which rather little is known.

It is to be hoped that this concept of sharing will go right through life. Wives may well have to fight a bit for proper priority for their husbands' attention and help with the children. If the average father was to be shut up at home with two or three children under seven, he would probably go bonkers. Yet he expects his wife to cope with all this and come up smiling with the supper. In addition, he may well get home late, tired, smelling slightly of drink and fall asleep in front of the telly. What's in all this for the woman?

Many of these battles are won or lost early in marriage and unless the woman gets her pound of flesh she may well be condemning herself to a somewhat lonely middle age, in which she is not doing much more than running a cut-price boarding house with an occasional holiday by the sea. I suggest, too, that wives should try and get as involved, directly and indirectly, in their husbands' work as is possible. Obviously, if the man does secret or confidential work, there may be areas of activity he cannot talk about, but I am always concerned by the man who says proudly, 'I never talk about work at home'. If he is a rather boring and limited businessman, what on earth is there left for him *to* talk about?

Money is another very delicate area if the wife stops working. There is nothing more humiliating for anyone, than to be totally dependent on someone else for money. Obviously, if the wife has no money and is not earning, she must have an allowance, but part of this must be regarded as hers, to do absolutely what she likes with—or she should retain reasonable access to the joint account. This was put to me very neatly the other day by a BBC producer who said 'The height—or the depth—of humiliation is to have to borrow the money for the *Tampax*.' This may sound a little crude when written baldly like this, but it does sum up what can become a desperate situation.

Having a Family

So far, I have assumed that a working wife will give up work at least until the children go to school, at which time, it may be possible to start part–time activity. We need also to consider briefly the possibility of going on work-ing. Under present economic conditions, this may become essential as it is often easier for a woman to retain a clerical, secretarial or teaching job than for a man to go on with factory work in a slump. In addition, the Equal Pay Act may possibly put pressure on employers to keep jobs open. Whether or not it is good for the family for mother to work is a difficult question but I suspect that a firm home base with her in charge is to be preferred, at least until school. One-parent families obviously come into a different category.

Although it is perfectly possible for a woman to go on working until late in pregnancy, and then go back to work, say a month later, I doubt if this is sensible and it would be very demanding. It is difficult to generalise, but probably one ought to aim at three to four months off work. Suitable arrangements must then be made to look after the children and this country is still deficient in the provision of day nurseries or crèches. On the Contin-ent, many factories provide highly sophisticated day nurseries with fully trained staff, in order to attract the right workers. Alternatively, private arrangements within the family or 'street group' can be made, but I ques-tion how satisfactory these are. One of the disadvantages of day nurseries, etc. is the problem of infection; it does mean that the young child will catch everything that goes, which can be a nuisance.

Going back to work may be essential, but the experts, with whom, for once, I agree, suggest that mum's best place is in the home, at least until nursery school. This can be boring, demanding and, indeed, frightening, but calm and balanced children are more likely to result from a stable home. Fathers can, and may increasingly play a part here. I recently took part in a TV discussion on which there was a splendid father who looked after the baby while his wife went out to work. What would help this situation is greater availability of part-time work at home. This requires imaginative organisation, but it is not impossible to achieve.

4.10

A mother with dependent young children is likely to be a difficult employee, because she must have time off for illness. And because she is likely to be over-stretched, her own health record may be disappointing. This could be an area of considerable social change over the next few years and we can watch its evolution with interest.

Middle Marriage

By now the children should be reaching adolescence and the career pattern established. Hopefully, as the children get to school, the wife will either get back to part-time work or develop activities outside the home. These are essential to give balance and interest to her life and to bring her into contact with other people. Otherwise she too will have nothing but domestic things to talk about and this is pretty boring for a tired husband. Although much is said about its virtues, I am unimpressed by the need for women to stay at and be devoted to home. The world is a big and exciting place and to remain human, they must be part of it. Over-devotion to domestic chores and standards is making an end out of a means, and this is dangerous.

Over the last ten years, I have been impressed by the number of quite sensible and competent men, who have had more problems from their teenage children than from their work. The relationship with the young may have gone by default and when there is a crisis they have no real contact on which to base a solution. In any case, it is unfair to leave it all to mum. But equally mum must see—and she does have some leverage—that dad carries his share of the load and actually does things with the children all the time and not just on holiday.

A few marriages end in disaster, often by coronary thrombosis, because the wife's ambition is greater than her husband's capacity. Such a wife will try and push her husband, by being demanding and dominating, further or faster than he was designed to go—and he will crack up. Many years ago, I did a pre-employment medical on a man who had had two coronaries and was trying to get a new and very demanding job. In agreement with the managing director of the operating company, I said 'no' and advised him about possible rehabilitation. His wife got hold of the chairman, got him the job and he was dead within a year.

Women need to realise that between a quarter and a third of them will land up as widows well before retiring age. Much of this is due to coronary thrombosis, which is, in my view, a disease largely related to the husband's way of life. They can see, as he gets older, that they do not overfeed him, that he takes a reasonable amount of exercise, takes his holidays and develops outside interests, etc. It is also quite important for a number of reasons that neither of them smoke cigarettes. How, for instance, can children be stopped from smoking, if one or both parents do? 'Don't do as I do, but do as I say' is a poor motto for bringing up the young.

A last point here, in the couple's fifties, is to begin thinking about retirement. Wives should nag their husbands into making proper provision for this. Such provision, which is fully described in M. Pilch (ed.), *The Retirement Book* (Hamish Hamilton, London), includes giving thought to activity, where to live, finance and health.

Late in Marriage

Marriage may be for better or for worse, but it is seldom for seven lunches a week. Unless properly planned for, retirement is 'work bereavement' and a retired man, who suddenly loses the status and identity of work, can go into a state of shock, from which he may die of a broken heart.

Retirement can be very like getting married all over again. The couple who may in fact have seen very little of each other, now have really to live in the house all the time. And the house has really to be lived in, which means that it has to be used, rather than kept tidy for occasional use, i.e. the wife has to change her attitude to what goes on in the home. Here again, I think that the husband should be encouraged to bear his share of the domestic load and do his share of the chores. By this time, the children having grown up, the wife should be well organised with her own outside interests and activities. Under no circumstances should she give them up to look after him. Make him get his own lunch and look after her for a change.

If the marital relationship has been poor or even just rather negative, the increased contact may put it under great strain. There could be a need for a great deal of fence-mending here. This demands a willingness to discuss problem areas freely and frankly without acrimony or fault-finding, coupled with a willingness to compromise and negotiate a new deal.

Poor Marriages

Life is quite difficult and demanding enough without the additional burden of a genuinely unhappy marriage. And there are plenty of these about.

4.12

Some incompatibility can be adjusted to and overcome by goodwill. But without this willingness to meet and discuss, these marriages drift on, either in nagging acquiescence or downright misery to one or both parties.

Now that divorce is both easier and more socially acceptable, I am strongly in favour of the termination of genuinely incompatible marriages. This is not to say that divorce should be made any easier or that marriage should be lightly undertaken on the grounds that it can be easily and simply terminated. I would rather see trial of marriage by cohabitation, than easy divorce—but this is a personal view, expressed, however, by one who had a second marriage.

Over the years of seeing people with what might loosely be called environmental difficulties, arising from miserable marriages, because of personality problems or just ordinary incompatibility, I have been impressed both by the improvement obtained by separation and the strength of a second marriage. Obviously in this the woman tends to get the worse of the deal because of her economic vulnerability, but she is to blame in at least half the cases and is usually just as unhappy as the man. Providing that she is reasonably provided for, I can see no reason for the perpetuation of misery.

There must, however, be one proviso to all this and that is the needs of the children. In this age of unstable and disturbed adolescents, parents having produced children, do have an obligation to give them a fair start from a stable base. On the whole, they should try and stick together, without obvious friction, until the young can stand on their own feet. Thereafter, they should try to stop everyone taking sides and try to set up new adult relations with the children.

It used to be thought that in nearly all circumstances, two parents were always better than one, no matter how disrupted the home. Opinions are now changing and there may be times when one stable parent is less disturbing for the child than tension and warfare. Clearly the parent, in one-parent families, has a desperately hard time—but it may be better in the end.

Working Wives

I have always taken the view that the woman who does two jobs has to be super-efficient to survive and do them both well. Running a home—even with good support from husband and family—and going out to work, demands a very precise assessment of priorities. Many women do, of course, achieve this, but in so doing, they must take great care to remain feminine and attractive. The mum-and-wife role must not be forgotten or there may well be disaster on one or other front. In the great majority of cases, work possibilities will be minimal while the children are young, but once they go to school and particularly if domestic help is available, the wife can get back to some work—and with both success and benefit.

There are a number of cases I know of, in which husband and wife either work for, or run the same organisation, although this obviously can be made to work I often wonder if it is really the best way round the course. Perhaps they either see too much of each other, or don't have enough else to talk about. It must also be pretty boring for the children. As has already been said, I am strongly in favour of women getting some activity outside the home, once the children do not need full-time attention.

I suspect that working couples have more difficulty in bringing up children than do others. The young need the right amount of attention and encouragement and very soon realise when they are being neglected. Similarly, there may be a tendency to have only one child, who may turn out to be undersized and precious, largely because he tends to be kept as an exhibit by his parents and not allowed to be a sentient individual in his own right. There used to be a feeling that 'only' children had serious disadvantages and tended to become neurotic, over-protected and too self-centred. Obviously this can happen, but with sensible up-bringing and great attention to friends, going off with peer groups etc., this can be overcome. In times of economic stress and over-population, there may be more to be said for the one-child family—but both parents and child are frightfully vulnerable if anything goes wrong.

The great thing, I believe, about having a working wife is that it will encourage the husband to pull his weight, appreciate his wife and not just sit back and expect to be looked after, unless, of course, the couple just rub along and mostly go their own ways—in which case the relationship might be worse still.

Childless Marriage

To start with a platitude; childless marriage can either be by design or accident. Usually it is only very self-centred (selfish) and insecure people, who refuse to have children. The ones that I know tend to rationalise their own emotional inadequacy by inventing reasons why they do not at least try to produce a family. There is no doubt that it is on the whole 'normal' to want to be succeeded and to produce something on which to lavish love and attention. Marriages without this need very careful attention to other points of focus if they are not to become either unbalanced or ludicrous.

4.14

About ten per cent of all marriages are childless or sub-fertile. We now know a great deal about this and many couples can be helped by expert investigation and treatment. Sub-fertility is usually a reflection of both parties, although one can also often say that it is either one or the other that is to blame. Clearly, if the man has a condition in which no sperm are produced, or get through, or the woman does not ovulate or has blocked fallopian tubes (which carry the egg cell to the womb), pregnancy is unlikely. The important thing here is to start investigation early and while fairly young (fertility falls off appreciably over the age of thirty) and to face the fact that both must be willing to be involved in the investigation, which can be trying and demanding. Mercifully the days in which women were operated on for their husbands' lack of sperm, have largely gone, but it did use to happen. If, after reasonable trial and treatment, there is still difficulty I am sure that the best thing is to stop trying. I know that this is much easier to say than to do, but any sub-fertile couple will tell you of the 'expectatory hell' that they go through every month, hoping for a pregnancy.

The best way round this is to consider adoption and this usually works out very successfully, although adopted children can be as disappointing and difficult as natural ones. The mere fact that this has been decided on stops the anxiety of expectation and the subsequent tranquility may lead to pregnancy. The trouble is, however, that adoption has become much more difficult; the abortion laws—which in my view must be kept liberal (no-one should have and no-one should be, an unwanted child)—and the bureaucrats, have made it very hard to provide suitable children, except possibly coloured ones from third world countries. If a couple can face the problems involved, this can be most gratifying and, in my limited experience, it seems to work.

Without children, a couple have to find other outlets and hopefully this should be more than lavishing on pets, the attention that would otherwise go on children. Childless wives should obviously have a serious and meaningful activity, preferably involving other people.

Unmarried Women

The unmarried woman has a range of difficult problems, which get worse as she gets older. Obviously she will be dedicated to her work and is likely to be career-minded. In practice, she may well be over-devoted to this and get a bit socially isolated or become overpowering or frightening. I once asked my very experienced 'boss' why a very attractive and competent middle-aged woman had never got married.

'That's easy,' he said, 'She must have been far too bossy when younger.'

Without going into detail, unmarried women have to solve the problem of what they do with their normal sexual drive, in their own way, by sublimation, by extra-marital relationships or by homosexual relationships. The latter seem easier for women than for their male counterparts, perhaps because the female relationship seems more inherently stable. Society is now mercifully much more tolerant of this type of liaison which can be lifelong and satisfying. The sexual problems of the unmarried woman can be solved, but the adjustment involved may be more difficult than in normal marriage.

Women, too, are exposed to all the pressures and temptations of over-indulgence and must guard against them in the same way as men. To a degree, they have to work to higher standards as they both fall harder and get branded more easily, i.e. a woman who is known to drink too much has a worse reputation than a similar man and is probably a greater social liability. Similarly, the girl who is 'easy to get' seems to finish up with a worse reputation than the bachelor who sleeps around. Life is hard and unfair.

The real crunch for an unmarried woman comes when she approaches retirement and then retires. Work has been her focus and great loneliness is her new bug-bear. Over-simplifying, she should, I believe, avoid becoming a fiercely militant independent spinster in 'tweeds and a thatched cottage,' but get involved, by conscious planning, in situations involving people. Obviously, if she has good family relationships, this is fine and now they really will be needed, but if not, and this tends to be the case, she must get herself into a social situation, perhaps with a housing group. In effect, she must go on working at something for as long as possible.

Working for a Woman

Although this booklet is about and for women, it would be unfair not to mention the 'male problem' when faced with a woman boss. The fact that, as supervisors, particularly at a younger age, women tend to be bad at dealing with each other, has already been referred to. It has also been suggested that mature women make more tolerant supervisors of the young. What has not been discussed, but is worth a brief mention for the sake of completeness, is the problem of the man reporting to a woman executive.

If a woman is going to survive in a man's world, an ability to cope with men will be one of the attributes of survival. If she does not have the managerial gift 'to manage', she is unlikely to make the top. But she will, of course, have to be tactful about this and her male colleagues will have to accept the hierarchical relationship as normal, as indeed they probably will and as they do in teaching and the civil service. Obviously, too, this is likely to become more common with the genuine development of equal pay and opportunity. The probability is that it will be the less competent men, with chips on their shoulders, who will actively resent a woman being promoted over them. If, on the other hand, a man has strayed into a woman's world, as may happen in agencies, or the rag trade, this is something he will have to live with as part of the job. Younger men still working their way up will almost certainly accept women over them, as part of the natural hierarchy. And, indeed, as time goes on and if more women remain in industry and commerce, the problem should become less.

The Last Years

It is a sad fact of life that women live longer than men, which means that most women will end their days as widows, often lonely and ill-provided for. About a third of them will be *prematurely* widowed, because their husbands die young—usually of a coronary thrombosis. This is a gloomy and complicated area involving both the adequacy of the social services and the community's attitude to the elderly. All that can be said here is that as this is a very real contingency, the possibility must be faced up to and adequate contingency planning undertaken. It is, for instance, silly to leave a frail old lady with a large Victorian house. Equally, a cantankerous granny can wreck a family of young children.

Some of the problems stem from the unwillingness of husbands to discuss money with their wives and others from a general reluctance to face unpleasant possibilities. I do believe, however, that older married couples should be brave enough to discuss what will happen if either of them 'fails to make the end of the week'.

Medical Problems

In spite of all the things that can, and do go wrong with their reproductive apparatus, women are tougher than men and live longer. Why this should be and quite what happens to women who work, rather than women who are housewives, we do not know.

Specific problems apart, women have to be careful, or sensible about the same hazards as men. As charm and attraction is perhaps a more important asset than to a man, women tend to be more disciplined about their weight and appearance, which is fine provided they do not waste too much money chasing the dictates of fashion and hobble about in shoes so silly that they walk like camels on hot bricks.

Drinking and smoking should be disciplined and indeed the latter abandoned: women might try taking more to cigars as a new fashion.

Similarly, reasonable physical fitness is equally important, so that regular exercise and bending and stretching routines for the more elderly are highly desirable. Group activities have a lot to commend them and it has been found, for both men and women that 'same age groups' are much better than having the young 'up-marketing the middle-aged'. Women should thus follow all the advice in the other three pamphlets in this series.

Sexuality

As has already been said, individuals must make up their own minds about the conditions under which they want to undertake sexual activity and this cannot be discussed here in detail. But they must, and now the great majority of them do, realise that unprotected sexual contact leads to pregnancy which has consequences far removed from the immediate sexual and emotional satisfaction. Alcohol lowers tolerance and removes common sense, so that many an unprotected girl is 'caught' at a party or led into an orgy of which she has little memory.

With the availability of the Pill and other reliable methods of contraception, there should now be no excuse for unwanted pregnancy. Nevertheless far too many unwanted pregnancies do still occur and, because it is (unfairly perhaps) the woman who suffers most, it must be up to her to see that she does not get 'caught'. Men, by running away, disappearing, or just being plain unhelpful, do manage to duck their responsibility and leave the woman to choose between an abortion or becoming an unmarried mother. And, as in the case of deserted wives, the law does not find it easy to extract maintenance from an unwilling father. What is essentially required is a much greater sense of responsibility and realisation of the consequences by both participants.

Young girls tend to succumb to the blandishments of older men, whose greater experience and promises lead to a false sense of security. Before the

4.18

war, a GP friend of mine worked near a large military barracks. When the girls came in frightened and pregnant, he used to say,

'Did he say it would be all right if you did it standing up?'
and mostly they said 'Yes', as this was a piece of local folklore.

Another danger to be guarded against is the chance of venereal or sexually transmitted disease, the risk of which is greater with casual liaisons or for businessmen away from home. Before embarking on such a relationship, it is worth both participants asking themselves the question: if he or she does this with me, who else might they have been with and is this likely to be all right? A simple contraceptive sheath protects against most of the hazards and may be a prudent investment.

Gynaecological Problems

From puberty to the menopause, a woman experiences a regular sequence of hormone-induced cyclical changes, which result in menstruation or the monthly period. These may be interrupted by pregnancy and lactation which produce another set of changes. Because her reproductive system is so complicated, it is not surprising that from time to time, it goes wrong or gives trouble. In addition, the vagina is a moist passage leading to the outside, so that it may easily become infected and cause minor but irritating symptoms.

Also, at the end of the reproductive cycle, a further set of changes, related to the cessation of ovulation and the run down of oestrogen production by the ovaries, occurs. This is known as the menopause or change of life. It is thus almost to be expected that most women will, at some time, have some minor upset or disease related to the changes in these systems. Most of them are minor, trivial and easily dealt with. It is, however, bad luck that most doctors are men, who are bored by these (usually minor) upsets, to which they then fail to devote the care and attention that is merited by the anxiety and inconvenience. The main 'organs' that cause trouble are the uterus or womb, its neck which protrudes into the vagina, the cervix, the ovaries which produce the egg cell and the vagina itself.

The object of the biological exercise is, of course, to produce a monthly egg cell which travels down the fallopian tubes into the womb. This has a special nutrient lining designed to nurture the fertilised ovum and see the foetus through pregnancy. If, as is nearly always the case, there is no fertilisation, the lining is not needed and has to be disposed of. Thus the monthly process of menstruation happens because the unused uterine lining, called the endometrium, has to be got rid of and replaced ready for the next chance of conception. The whole cycle is under hormone control which starts in the pituitary, a small organ at the base of the brain, and is mainly reflected by the intermittent production of progesterone and oestrogen by the ovaries. If conception occurs, the whole system changes gear, there is no monthly period and the growing foetus is accepted and nurtured by the uterus. At the same time the breasts are, again under hormone control, prepared for lactation. Once pregnancy is over, the cycle settles down again and proceeds more or less regularly until the next pregnancy or the menopause.

As every girl knows, there is a close connection between the hormone system and the emotions. Anxiety, ill-health and other events can upset the cycle and cause fear of pregnancy. Within ten days or so of pregnancy being established, the hormone change is reflected in the hormone content of the urine. This forms the basis of the rapid pregnancy tests now generally available.

Expelling the menstrual flow can be a painful process especially if the cervical canal is tight or the flow contains clots or lumps of debris. The muscular uterus has to squeeze all this out, which may result in colicky pain. An easy cure for this may be to stretch or dilate the cervical canal and scrape out the inside of the uterus. This is known as dilation and curettage and is the basis of early abortion procedures (up to three months) and diagnostic curettage to establish the cause of bleeding or uterine enlargement.

Menstruation is obviously an emotive subject to which a lot of behavioural folklore has been attached. Mercifully it is now considered much more sensibly, with the probability that it causes less minor discomfort. But there is no doubt that some people do get painful periods and if these cannot be dealt with by simple pain-killers, they ought to be medically investigated. There is neither excuse nor reason for regular invalidism in relation to what is a normal and natural process.

The monthly cycle does have effects or manifestations beyond the uterus. Thus there is the condition of pre-menstural tension with discomfort, irritability and perhaps some emotional instability, as well as possibly painful swelling of the breasts. Some of this is again to be expected, but if it is significantly limiting, it should be investigated and thought about. Because of the hormone cycle, there is a tendency to water-logging of the tissues, towards the end of the cycle. This can cause painful breasts, swollen ankles and gain in weight.

The Pill which is primarily designed to stop ovulation and fertilisation, by interfering with the hormone cycle, also has the effect of smoothing out or regularising the cycle. It is thus also used for treatment as well as contraception. There are, in fact, several different types of Pill with their own

4.20

indications and contra-indications. They also have side-effects which if not often serious, do require monitoring and supervising. Taking the Pill, often for years, should always be under expert supervision and subject to periodic review. It is a powerful weapon which acts by altering a natural process and although it is probably the most reliable and convenient contraceptive, it cannot and should not be taken light-heartedly or without proper advice. It is also worth remembering that not all Pills suit all people and it is sensible to find the right one for you, if necessary by trying more than one. Mainly it is the oestrogen content that causes the side-effects and the withdrawal of this, by stopping after so many days, that produces a blood flow which is in fact a pseudo-menstruation.

The Menopause or Change of Life

Fertility or the ability to reproduce is much more finite in women than it is in men. Indeed, several years before ovulation ceases it is regarded as unwise for women to become pregnant, i.e. having a baby at forty is much more hazardous than at twenty or even thirty.

What happens is that somewhere between forty-five and fifty (or there-abouts) the hormone control system runs down and menstruation becomes irregular, scantier and finally ceases altogether. The run-down period can vary from a few months to over a year. Unfortunately, and largely because of the associated hormone upset, there are other symptoms, such as hot flushing, which can be very embarrassing and a degree of quite severe emotional lability.

Clearly too, the menopause is related to other emotional changes and fears. To a degree, it marks the end of 'being a woman' or at least is thought so to do. As, at about the same time, women are facing middle age, and the readjustments that this involves, the menopause has become the dumping ground for a host of minor and major symptoms relating more to general discontent and uncertainty, than to any inherent change. In my view, much backache etc. in women is due to psychosomatic causes rather than gynae-cology or bone and joint disease. It is a manifestation of dis-ease rather than disease, and should be treated as such.

The menopause thus does present a range of problems and need for adjustment, but many of the symptoms can and should be treated, largely by hormone replacement. Some doctors may be unsympathetic and dis-inclined to give the necessary consideration. Luckily there is now a development of special menopause clinics where these things can be better dealt with. There is also a current fashion to postpone the menopause by oestrogen replacement therapy. The thought here is not only to deal with the symptoms but also to postpone the other associated changes, like putting on a bit of weight and becoming rounder in the buttocks. It is too soon to make a final judgement on this, but certainly symptoms should be treated.

Women tend to think that the menopause also marks the end of the sex life. This is nonsense. All that happens is that they can no longer become pregnant. The relief of this anxiety should add greater enjoyment rather than diminution. It is wise, however, to go on taking contraceptive precautions until twelve periods have been missed. Provided both partners want it, sexual activity can go on late into life, i.e. well after sixty in some cases. Problems arise when one partner 'tails off' before the other and then feels guilty and inadequate. In practice, this may happen to the man rather than the woman. I suspect that fatigue, particularly in men, is often a limiting factor and sometimes a holiday, or general letting up can be a help. Should there be a problem, it must be faced and discussed, possibly with an expert, with honesty and frankness.

Inevitably, too, an element of boredom can creep into sexual activity after many years of marriage and in middle age there may be a tendency to adventure and change. One cannot dogmatise about this, but women do have an opportunity to keep themselves attractive and 'different' and should give considerable thought as to how change can be introduced. For instance, there is no need to confine intercourse to the end of the day when one is tired: mornings at week-ends can be better than late at night. The situation can, of course, arise where tired and guilty men are driven to demonstrate their virility in a promiscuous way and this can lead to traumatic if not tempestuous affairs with younger women. There is also, the psychologists say, a tendency for undemonstrative women, married to obsessional business men, to drive them in the same direction because of their coldness.

Gynaecological Symptoms

The main symptom is bleeding. Any vaginal bleeding which occurs in younger people between periods, or in older people after they have stopped, must be treated seriously. Similarly, heavy or prolonged periods leading to anaemia should be investigated, because the cause of the bleeding, which may be a simple fibroid tumour as well as the loss itself, needs treatment.

4.22

Bleeding

This comes either from the lining of the uterus or from benign or malignant growths of the womb or cervix. Most of the causes are benign and the results of treating the malignant ones are excellent if done early enough. Cancer of the cervix is detected by the cervical smear, facilities for which are now available countrywide. Because of this, the death rate from this condition is beginning to fall.

As has been said, all bleeding must be investigated, usually by a dilation and curettage (D and C), which is a simple procedure involving, at most, a couple of nights in hospital.

Hysterectomy

Further treatment may then involve removal of the womb—Hysterectomy. This is not usually a serious operation and most patients leave hospital in ten to fourteen days. But sadly it is still an emotive procedure which symbolically destroys 'womanhood', so that full recovery and readjustment takes much longer than it should. Except in young people, for whom the operation is indicated for serious reasons, what is being done is to remove a piece of worn-out, damaged and no longer useful equipment. Prolonged heavy periods for instance, can cause considerable long-term disability, but are immediately cured by surgery.

Psychological aspects apart, there is no hardship and immense gain from hysterectomy; sexual activity should be completely normal and if the vagina is a bit dry, this can be overcome by a simple lubricant like KY jelly. In fact, hysterectomy can be one of the most successful gynaecological operations. In relation to the operation, there is a technical problem as to whether or not to remove the ovaries as well as the womb. After the menopause, this does not matter, but earlier, their removal will produce a premature menopause. Leaving them behind however, retains the cyclical pattern without the possibility of menstruation and this can cause problems, particularly of tension, etc. But the moral of all this, is that women, childbearing possibilities apart, should be keen, rather than reluctant to have a hysterectomy, to relieve them of damaging symptoms and the possibility of cancer.

In another group of conditions, the supports of the uterus may be weakened, usually by childbirth. The uterus then drops and may even protrude. Not only is this inconvenient and uncomfortable, it may also interfere with bladder control. This is called prolapse and is again simply dealt with surgically.

Sterilisation

Partly because of the population explosion and partly for common-sense

4.23

reasons, there has been, over the past decade a growing acceptance of sterilisation as a permanent method of contraception. If, in a man, the tube which leads from the testicle, called the *vas deferens*, is cut on both sides, the man becomes sterile. The operation—vasectomy—is simple to do as an out-patient and under local anaesthetic. In India, for instance, the facility is offered behind screens on railway stations, as a method of population control. Sterilising a woman by blocking or cutting the fallopian tubes is more complicated and may involve an abdominal operation, although there are other ways of doing it. Both procedures are meant to be permanent, but there are possibilities, in skilled hands, of rejoining the cut tubes in both men and women.

For mature people, over the age of forty, perhaps, who have had three children, or for younger people with large families or inheritable diseases, this can be a good way of permanently relieving the anxiety of further pregnancy. It is not easy to decide who should be sterilised and due thought must be given to the fact that circumstances and inclinations may alter, marriages may be upset by death or divorce, and so on. As the woman's productive life is so much more circumscribed than the man, she is giving up less, as it were, by having this terminated ten years early, at a time when she is in many cases too old to start or add to a family. But the operation is simpler and cheaper for the man, who may be equally relieved by having his fertility curtailed. In either case, it is a difficult decision which must be freely discussed and agreed by both parties before a conscientious doctor will perform the operation. With the permission of both parties, it is a perfectly legal procedure.

Vasectomy clinics are now common in this country and will certainly continue to grow. In neither case should there be any interference with sexual function, although unexpected psychological upset can and does rarely occur. In practice, sterilisation is often a sensible procedure, which ought perhaps to be considered more often. It could turn out to be safer than years on the Pill. Certainly, marriages which are haunted by the fear of further pregnancy are enormously helped by sterilisation and it may be essential on eugenic grounds.

Vaginal Infections

As has already been implied, the vagina is a moist passage which communicates freely with the exterior. For both these and other reasons, it can be very prone to minor infections. These mostly cause irritation, discharge or leakage, and some anxiety. A common cause of infection can be a retained foreign body, like a forgotten vaginal tampon which becomes infected and causes discharge and irritation. Such neglect can be embarrassing, even if the cure is dramatic. Because of its 'geography', it is not easy to disinfect

4.24

the vagina so that the effective treatment of infections can be tedious and difficult. It is perhaps unfortunate for women who are genuinely bothered by minor gynaecological complaints, that most doctors are men, who may be somewhat disinclined to treat them with the consideration they deserve. In such cases, the woman must peg away and demand proper consideration, possibly from a specialised clinic or Family Planning Centre.

Venereal Disease

Gonorrhoea and syphilis, the traditional venereal diseases in this country, are transmitted by sexual intercourse. Both diseases are eminently treatable in skilled hands and indeed demand instant investigation. The infection can only be acquired from an infected partner, who was in turn infected by a third person. Thus VD tends to be acquired from extra-marital liaisons and then, perhaps tragically, passed on into the marriage.

Obviously, a promiscuous woman has much greater chances of infecting several men, but equally any woman may be infected by a man who has active disease: one of the problems is that the symptoms are much more apparent in the man, who gets pain, discharge, irritation, etc. A highly infectious woman may have virtually no symptoms and indeed be unaware of being infected or infectious. Thus it may be the man who gets caught and may then infect his wife. Clearly, however, in dealing with an infectious disease like this, the doctors must be able to follow up and treat all the contacts.

Treatment of VD is now relatively easy and effective, although penicillin-resistant strains of gonorrhoea and syphilis are not uncommon. Men tend to get mildly dramatic symptoms—as well as feeling guilty—and come for treatment. It is the woman who does not realise that she is infected who provides the reservoir of the disease.

Strictly speaking, any disease that is transmitted by sexual contact can be regarded as venereal, but in practice the term is confined to gonorrhoea and syphilis in this country and one or two other ones in tropical countries. They are all conditions which have long-term, serious effects on the afflicted. Gonorrhoea, for instance, can cause sterility in women and urinary obstruction in men, whereas syphilis, in what is called its late stage, has disastrous effects on the nervous system in both men and women.

Over the last twenty-five years, a new group of conditions involving urinary or urethral infection in men has been isolated. Obviously when the symptoms present, the first thought is of traditional VD, but when this has been ruled out, search for other infective agents begins. This group of infections, called *non-specific urethritis*, comes either from a virus infection, or by the man becoming infected by organisms—like the Trichomonas—which commonly cause minor vaginal infections in his wife. Thus, in the

4.25

normal course of married life, the infection gets shuttled backwards and forwards. Treatment obviously involves both partners and can be tedious. As with all infections, unprotected intercourse should not occur until the infection is fully under control. This condition is not now uncommon and absolutely no social stigma attaches to it—although until everyone is reassured, it is mixed up inevitably with the 'guilt' of possible VD and suspicion of extra-marital liaison by either party.

Painful Intercourse (Dyspareunia)

Conditions in the vagina or its outlet, or sometimes within the pelvis, but pressing on the vagina, can cause pain and discomfort during intercourse. Similarly, vaginal infections, which may produce an inflamed surface with even slight bleeding, will inevitably be uncomfortable. Full recovery from a gynaecological operation may be delayed several months until the scar tissue in the vagina is completely healed.

Psychological upsets, with fear or guilt about sex (often related to childhood experience) and general tension, can also make intercourse difficult for a woman. Obviously, if the vagina goes into spasm or the whole area tightens up, penetration cannot take place. Rather similarly the persistance of a thick hymen can cause difficulty.

Most of these conditions—either physical or psychological—are amenable to expert treatment. Really all that is required is for the woman to be prepared to seek advice and discuss the situation frankly; not all doctors are good at this, but most family planning centres and gynaecological departments, provide a special service and a frank no-nonsense atmosphere.

Breast Surveillance

Up until very recently, we British have been reluctant to face the possibility of having cancer because of its sinister reputation as a 'killer'. In point of fact, about half the cancers seen by doctors are successfully treated. As to the other half, the results of treating many of them could be dramatically improved if only the patient would present—or come to the doctor—with the earliest symptoms. Because of the inherent, but still lingering fear of cancer, patients, particularly women, tend to put off going to the doctor until it may be too late.

Any unusual swelling or lump, bleeding, area of pain, or change in normal routine—like bowel habit, digestion or appetite, particularly in older people—should be investigated as a matter of urgency. Cancers start as a circumscribed growth and, provided they can be technically removed, the chances of cure are then excellent. Cancer is so called, because it is from the Greek 'crab', which implies that it spreads sideways. Once a cancer has spread locally, by infiltration, or been carried further round the

4.26

body via the blood or lymphatic systems, the outlook is much worse, because the spread cannot be reached so easily by surgery or X-ray.

All this is particularly true of breast cancer, which is the biggest single killer of middle-aged women. And it is only relatively recently, that the results of treating it have begun to improve. Once the cancer has spread beyond the breast (usually first to the glands in the axilla), the five-year cure rate, which is the way in which cancer treatment is assessed, drops to about thirty per cent, but if removed early, the cure rate can be as high as ninety per cent, and the smaller the growth, the less the amount of breast tissue that has to be removed. Early treatment is thus dramatically successful and delay disastrous. When I was a student, and then when I was back in hospital again after the war, we still used to see ladies with large and obvious lumps in their breasts coming to the out-patients. They must have known about the lump for a considerable time, but were obviously frightened to come up to hospital, or to their doctor, because of the fear of cancer.

Apart from the skin, or perhaps in the mouth, no part of the body is more accessible than the breast. We now know that it is only by early and expert examination that the smallest lumps can be found and dealt with.

Four processes are essential to success:

1. The woman's willingness to face the fact that she might have cancer and to *do* something about it at once. The more all this is discussed and brought out into the open, the easier it will be. A friend of mine who runs a 'cancer clinic' in Chicago had a waiting list of 650 women for breast screening, thanks to the publicity following Mrs Ford and Mrs Rockefeller.
2. Expert clinical examination.
3. An infra-red scan called 'Thermovision', which is totally painless and picks up hot areas in the breast which might be suspicious.
4. A special soft tissue X-ray called a mammogram, which may even reveal 'suspicious areas' too small to feel.

If anything suspicious is found as a result of any or all of these procedures, the next step is usually to do a small local operation to remove the area and examine it under a microscope. This is the only way in which the diagnosis can be made—either positively or negatively. The operation, called a biopsy, can be done as an out-patient, but it is often better to stay in for a couple of days.

With luck this removal may be all that is necessary, otherwise, more extensive removal may be required as a second and later procedure. The days of large mutilating operations, involving total removal of the breast and underlying muscle, known as radical mastectomy, have now largely gone. Mostly what is called 'lumpectomy' is done, or failing this, local removal of the whole breast, simple mastectomy, which although frightening, is not in itself a serious operation. At a later date, it is now often possible to restore the contour by plastic surgery and the use of implants. To follow the treatment though, once the scar has healed, there should be no pain or disability and full restoration of arm and shoulder function is to be expected. In some cases it may be necessary to follow the operation with a course of X-ray therapy, to deal with any possible spread, but this is not done so often now as a routine. Obviously, it is embarrassing to be lop-sided and have only one bosom and, of course, this takes getting used to by both husband and wife. But the effects are psychological rather than physical and it is a small price to pay for a cancer cure. BUPA has a film on 'Screening for Breast Cancer'—screening is the name given to the presumptive search for unsuspected disease (see Booklet 1)—and this film closes with a sequence of a woman who teaches children to swim, diving into a swimming pool in a two-piece bathing costume. She had had her breast removed, but retained full charm and function with the aid of a special bra.

Attendance for a cervical smear has now become an accepted part of our national life and clinics or centres are freely available. Breast screening is the new growth point in preventive medicine and we hope that it will not be too long before there is a similar countrywide network for it. Currently, we in BUPA have three such centres and we find about eight cancers per 1000 women seen, which makes this a very rewarding activity. About twelve per cent have to have biopsies, but the great majority are sent away reassured and happy, having faced the possibility and come out with a clean bill. Of course, we are not yet clever enough to win, or be right all the time, but this is a very great step forward in treating a major scourge which kills 30,000 women a year in this country.

Notwithstanding all the modern technology, the most important part of the screening is to learn systematic self-examination of the breast. Having been taught this, the woman should carry it out regularly every month. In the end, it is *by knowing the way round her own breasts*, and then reporting any change, that early diagnosis becomes practicable. American experience has shown that once indoctrinated and motivated, it is the women themselves who detect the very early lumps and present them for treatment. Although bosoms can vary greatly in consistency and size, it is easy to learn what are normal painful areas, lumps, etc. and be taught which ones matter and which ought to be removed. Once this skill has been acquired, it can be used for the rest of life, when, hopefully, death will be from another cause, or just old age.

The last point to make is that not all lumps in the breast are cancerous; in

4.28

fact, more are benign than malignant. Similarly, not all discharge from the nipple means a sinister growth. There are benign small lumps and larger cysts containing fluid, both of which are harmless. But once any abnormal area has been found, it must be removed, either by suction through a needle or by operation. The only place for breast lumps is under the microscope after local removal. But because of the risk, all lumps must be regarded as serious until they have been proved otherwise.

Readers: do please remember that at the moment breast cancer is to women, much what coronary thrombosis is to men—a major and, hopefully, preventable cause of death. Much of the remedy lies in your own hands and every husband would prefer a live, but possibly lop-sided wife to being a widower. Please learn and carry out regular examination and attend one of the special clinics if there is one in your area. If not, demand that one should be established.

As I have said, there is a thirty-minute film and also an illustrated booklet (*Breast Cancer*) available from BUPA. If you want any further help or advice, do please write to the Women's Unit at the BUPA Medical Centre (Webb House, 210 Pentonville Road, King's Cross, London N1 9TA) and we will try to help. Women themselves made the NHS provide the cervical smear; they should, in my view, now do the same for breast screening. The provision of facilities is now improving and the NHS has several pilot schemes running. The Royal Marsden Hospital in London and the Queen Elisabeth Hospital in Newcastle under Dr Stark also have 'Well Woman Centres'. All of these will advise as to the nearest source of help.

Conclusion

This is being written in International Women's Year at a time when equality of pay and opportunity are becoming more of a reality. But it is in equality of domestic and social relations that women have the most to gain. They are seemingly tougher than men and certainly live longer. Our current social behaviour makes it difficult for the average middle-aged woman to get back into the circulation she enjoyed before she was married. Basically, the remedy lies in her own hands: she must demand a more equal role in the home and come back into the world with more confidence. By having more worthwhile things to do she is likely to avoid boredom, backache and the dis-ease that currently leads her to haunt the doctor's surgery with nebulous aches and pains.

Having, on the whole, persuaded the male world to give them legal equality, women will have to learn to live with the consequences. This basically means becoming self-sufficient in middle and older age—and not feeling too strongly that the world owes them a living.

In this respect, attitudes towards the consequences of easier divorce will have to be faced. Although I am in favour of this, I freely admit that it may well bear harder on the middle-aged woman than the man, who, as a minimum, has more economic options. The law is moving in favour of a better settlement for the wife, but unless she gets back into circulation, inevitably she is going to be lonely. As for the lonely elderly, we are still very much in the phase of developing community support mechanisms, and one of the answers is to try to encourage them to live in non-institutional groups.